DIET RIGHT FOR YOUR
PERSONALITY TYPE

DIET RIGHT FOR YOUR
PERSONALITY TYPE

THE REVOLUTIONARY 4-WEEK WEIGHT-LOSS PLAN THAT WORKS FOR **YOU**

JEN WIDERSTROM

HARMONY
BOOKS · NEW YORK

Published in the United States by Harmony Books, an imprint of the Crown Publishing Group, a division of Penguin Random House LLC, New York.
crownpublishing.com

Harmony Books is a registered trademark, and the Circle colophon is a trademark of Penguin Random House LLC.

Library of Congress Cataloging-in-Publication Data
Names: Widerstrom, Jen, author.
Title: Diet right for your personality type : the revolutionary 4-week weight-loss plan that works for you / Jen Widerstrom.
Description: New York : Harmony Books, [2017] | Includes bibliographical references.
Identifiers: LCCN 2016039328| ISBN 9780451497987 (hardback) | ISBN 9780451497994 (ebook)
Subjects: LCSH: Weight loss. | Personality. | Self-care, Health. | BISAC: HEALTH & FITNESS / Diets. | HEALTH & FITNESS / Weight Loss. | SELF-HELP / Motivational & Inspirational.
Classification: LCC RM222.2 .W45233 2017 | DDC 613.2/5—dc23 LC record available at https://lccn.loc.gov/2016039328

ISBN 978-0-451-49798-7
Ebook ISBN 978-0-451-49799-4

Printed in the United States of America

Illustrations by Ben Ceccarelli
Recipe contribution by Laney Schwartz of Life Is but a Dish
Jacket design by Jennifer Carrow
Jacket photograph by the Riker Brothers

10 9 8 7 6 5 4 3 2 1

First Edition

I dedicate this book to you . . . because you deserve it.

CONTENTS

INTRODUCTION

have a confession. And I'm probably the last person you expect to admit this, but it needs to be said before you read anything else in this book: exercise and diet are not what they appear to be. In fact, I'd argue that most exercise and diet programs are mostly *unhealthy*.

Not what you were expecting, huh? Before you think I've lost my mind, I'm not saying exercise itself is harmful or that most diets will make you sick. The pertinent issue, as I see it, is how you implement these weight-loss programs into your life.

If you don't understand why you eat well (or not well)—and how the answers can be different *every day*—then you are setting yourself up for failure. This is what happens with almost every diet plan. One failure leads to another, and then the next thing you know, you believe that you can't change your body or your life. This is the vicious cycle that leads to weight gain, a lack of courage and confidence, and never-ending frustration.

But I can simplify the process, removing the downfalls of other diets, and put you in control of your body. How? By pointing out the one issue that every diet plan consistently refuses to address: *you.*

The problem with most diet books is that they don't acknowledge, recognize, or give power to how all of us are beautifully different and complex. Your individuality should be celebrated as a competitive *advantage*. And that's exactly what I'm going to show you how to do. Instead of feeling bad about your past obstacles and defeats when it comes to losing weight, I will show you how to elevate your unique qualities as strengths—how to use them in order to achieve success.

So before you start one more program destined to fail, it's time to reveal how diet and fitness really work. Just think about it for a moment. Strip away the 101 superfoods, the latest trends, and even your pretenses surrounding any gym environment and think about how you, or I, or anyone else functions on a daily basis.

We all have good and bad days. Are the reasons you eat healthy on the good days going to be the same as what knocks you off track (or keeps you on track) on the bad ones? What about the willpower it takes to avoid every dessert in your pantry on those tough days? Or the strength it takes not to let the defeating conversation in your head win? We know that these difficult situations pose different problems. And how we approach them is often different and based on our personality traits. Yet these are the aspects of health and weight loss that we never discuss.

How can you build a plan for your life when you're not considering *your life*? You need to examine how your personality—the unique characteristics and DNA that make you *you*—are the most important part of the journey of losing weight and living the life you want.

That's why I wrote this book. I'm tired of seeing failure. My work with clients has proven to me that the answer isn't just in the foods you eat or the workout you choose—it's in you. In the uniqueness that makes you *you*: your personality. *Diet Right for Your Personality Type* is a breakdown of five core personality types that I've discovered in my time helping to transform thousands of lives. These personalities are as follows:

- The critical-thinking **Organized Doer**
- The outgoing **Swinger**
- The free-spirited **Rebel**
- The selfless **Everyday Hero**
- The strong-minded **Never-Ever**

They are based on the five dominant personalities I've seen in more than a decade of working with my clients—the specific characteristics that can be strengths (or weaknesses) when it comes to succeeding on your weight-loss plan. And my four-week program is designed to work with each personality type to capitalize on its core characteristics and give you every advantage when it comes to losing the weight once and for all.

But this program is much more than just self-identification. It's about finally understanding why one-size-fits-all solutions have never worked for you in the past, and how you can use your own personality traits to thrive on the perfect plan, a plan created just for your type.

Each person needs an individualized program of diet and exercise—one that honors the individual and his or her personality—to inspire success. A diet has to be geared toward your personality to really work for you. I'm sure you've seen this in your own life: what worked for your best friend or someone in your family didn't work for you. Personality traits must be taken into account for anyone to succeed on a diet and ultimately keep weight off.

What is "personality," anyway?

I think of personality like a puzzle. You are made up of hundreds of different pieces that make up "you" as a whole. Each puzzle piece is a distinctive and enduring aspect of your personality—what motivates you, the way you think and act, and typical patterns of behavior you've had most of your life. Many of those pieces apply to your actions and reactions, to how you eat, how you diet, and even how you approach exercise.

Pause and take a look around an everyday lunch environment, and you'll see what I mean.

When you have lunch with your sister, for example, you can predict what she'll order—she eats the exact same thing at the exact same times every day. That's because she's motivated by order and organization. She knows she needs more nutritional variety, but it's so much more comfortable to stick to routine. She has the personality type I call "The Organized Doer."

Your co-worker is the total opposite. You don't know what he'll order because he loves the adventure of eating. As "The Swinger," he is happiest when trying something new—he gets fired up by the novelty of things—even if they might be fattening. He's always trying the latest diet, too, and his weight seems to go up and down.

When your best friend tries a strict or inflexible diet, she usually has trouble following through. Why? Because her personality type is "The Rebel," and most plans are far too detail oriented and restrictive for her. She'd rather not commit to dieting, so she will be deciding her lunch on the fly . . . that is, when she eventually has lunch. As usual, for any set plans, she's running late.

Few things mean more to your mother than friends and family, and she loves connecting with them around a great meal. That's why she's always game for a lunch date, plus she otherwise may not make time for herself to eat! She is like a lot of us, a true "Everyday Hero": she puts herself too far down the priority list, and her own nutrition and fitness always suffer as a result.

Finally, there's your neighbor. Intelligent but detached from healthy choices with a "why even try" attitude. I've worked with lots of people like this—fantastic, successful individuals, but when it comes to dieting and exercising, their mind-set is, "What's the point of trying? I'll probably fail anyway." I call this personality type "The Never-Ever."

Your friends and family, and really all of us, fit into one of my five personality types. I've found that understanding these types and how they apply to your life is the secret to weight-loss success.

In this book, I'll help you identify and understand what type of approach will best match your dominant personality traits and lifestyle. From there, I will help you personalize it to your needs by supplying a tailored road map for losing weight, eating nutritiously, and getting (and staying) in ideal shape. I've designed an individualized four-week program based on each personality type that holds the secret to fat-burning, increased energy, faster metabolism, better health, and emotional peace.

Each plan has been designed to work with the traits that dominate each personality. For example, for "The Organized Doer" who thrives on structure, I've designed a plan that will tell you exactly what, when, and how to eat, but if you are "The Swinger," that plan won't work for you because you're too adventurous and will become bored if you don't have options. So "The Swinger" plan offers a weekly menu with an array of food choices and more decision-making freedom.

No matter which personality type you are, with my plan you can expect to drop pounds every single week. You'll learn to outsmart the eating patterns that have blocked you in the past and make eating an enjoyable (and effective) experience. This program will transform your relationship with food, I promise. When it comes down to it, this program will empower you to take control of your life and your personality type, once and for all.

Understanding your personality, and what specifically makes you tick, is the X factor when it comes to having the mind-set you need to succeed on any weight-loss plan. The problem with most diet books is that they do not honor the individual. They overlook the uniqueness in all of us—when we really should be celebrating that individuality. We can push through any personal obstacles because we view our unique qualities as strengths.

When given the tools to succeed, you'll thrive, witnessing how even the smallest victories can and will morph into huge accomplishments. Not only does my program simplify the process by offering the clear advice and support that you need—including the eating plans, recipes, exercises, and more—but it also removes stress because it feels so much more natural, as it's specifically tailored to your individual needs.

With this book, I've taken all the guesswork out of what will work for your body. And all you need to do is follow my advice, and watch your body change for the better.

Unlike most books, *Diet Right for Your Personality Type* will not become useless in four weeks. I'm here to teach you how to adapt to any scenario because the program is customized to your way of thinking and being. No matter what is going on in your life, this plan will have a stabilizing effect on you and deliver a realistic plan that is proven to work, along with the lasting results you've always wanted.

MY STORY

If you're going to let me into your life, it's only fair that I let you into mine. I've seen the physical and emotional pain that stems from weight gain in individuals, couples, and families. I've had my own ups and downs in life, so I will share my story, hoping it renews your belief in your own.

My story begins as a little girl with crooked bangs and a crooked smile to match. Emotional, shy, but extremely loved, I was a handful from the get-go. My parents, Norm and Lynn, married forty-three years now, were both educators and coaches at high schools in the Chicago suburbs. My siblings and I were raised on a steady diet of work ethic, integrity, honesty, and family. We ate dinner together every night, were encouraged to ask questions, and were always supported to pursue whatever we wanted to go after.

From a young age, I loved gymnastics and ended up training at it for more than ten years. During high school, I expanded on my love of sports and participated in track and diving. When it was time to graduate, my parents supported my ambition to experience new surroundings, and I attended the University of Kansas to pursue a degree in sports administration. Once again, sports were at the forefront of my life. I was a walk-on (nonscholarship) member of the rowing team initially, but ultimately I switched over to track and field. What started as another walk-on experience ended in a complete transformation, and by my senior year I became a national-level competitor in the NCAA and the best female hammer thrower in school history.

A funny thing happened, though, that I did not expect. If you asked me, "Who are you?" leading up to my college graduation, my answer was clear:

"I'm a Division One athlete in the Big Twelve Conference—team captain, record holder—a leader in the student-athlete committee, all while pursuing a degree in sports administration."

My identity was intact and my list of projects and accomplishments made me feel worthy and important. But just one month after graduation, I had nothing to say. It was the strangest, emptiest feeling. I didn't have anything going on that made me feel like I mattered. I was bartending in my hometown and had no idea what was next. I felt such a loss of identity and loss of value because I didn't know what I had to offer.

I also started to struggle with my relationship with food and exercise. Up to this point, I had always been an athlete who executed my workouts and meals for performance-based results. I never had to worry about how many calories I ate because we trained several hours a day in college. I would literally have an entire Chipotle burrito and still want more, so without hesitation I would just pop back in line and order another one. I would do the same with finishing off entire pizzas and baskets and baskets of bread or chips.

The volume of my food was out of control but, again, I had no idea that it was because I was so active that it never showed up on the scale. You can imagine my surprise when just a few months after I graduated—continuing to eat as I did in college, but at a fraction of the activity level—my weight shot up.

It was "only" ten to fifteen pounds, but it happened so quickly and really was my first wake-up call to making a change. What was more disturbing to me than my weight was how I felt every day. No energy, no drive, no confidence.

I knew action was needed, but I didn't know what to do. Naturally, I looked to my peers and popular health magazines to help me lose weight. My friend went to the gym first thing in the morning, and even though I hated getting up that early, I asked to join her, but I never made it. Every time my alarm would go off, I would hit snooze for more than an hour, then bury myself in guilt for missing the workout. Ultimately, my desire to work out in the morning (a healthy intention) became a very unhealthy behavior because it triggered negative emotions. Missing the workouts made me angry at myself, then led to a bad day of eating because I felt like I was a failure.

No matter what I did, though, nothing made a difference for me; I only felt worse after every attempt and failure. Looking back now, I see that I was blindly doing what was working for *others* without taking into account what would actually work for *me*.

For example, I remember reading an article about the benefits of Greek yogurt, so I started eating it daily. I was choking it down, though, because the truth is, I'm a very picky eater and I hated the yogurt! I would never finish it and always felt unsatisfied after breakfast, which ultimately led to my being famished by lunchtime, leading to more bad food choices. And so the cycle continued: trying something that was working for someone else, not seeing results myself, and feeling like a failure, which led to guilt, which led to bad choices.

This was my life. Struggling with my self-image, my eating, my fitness. Following the plans that seemed to work for others but didn't work for me. It may sound a lot like your life—and we have more in common than you think.

CLARITY AND REINVENTION

My struggle made me stronger and led to the biggest breakthrough of my life. For the first time I allowed myself to fully be myself. Just Jen! I stopped trying to be like everyone else and allowed my decisions each day to reflect my truest, happiest self. *All* of this began through my personalizing my choices surrounding food and exercise and the way they affected my health and self-esteem—this was the catalyst that brought my true self to the surface and continues to be the basis of my success today.

After years of failure, I realized that I needed to honor what was best for the real me to be successful. Why was I eating foods I hated and following a routine that didn't jive with my life and my personality? And why did I think that doing what I hated was going to result in success? I needed to follow a plan that suited *me*—suited my personality, my likes and dislikes. I needed a plan customized for me.

I began to make my breakfasts and dinners for the week in advance; otherwise I'd be skipping the most important meal of the day and then eating cheese and crackers for dinner. I also stopped leaving home without a snack stashed in my purse and a big bottle of water to keep me honest through long unpredictable days. And finally, I began training with a workout buddy to help motivate me and get me through the doors of my gym consistently.

This shift in mind-set changed everything. Not only was I seeing results on the scale, but I also felt an empowered change in myself. I was listening to myself versus looking outward to others. It changed the way I felt about myself as a woman—in conversations, in dating, and in what I offered the world.

After I found work as a fitness model for a huge nutrition company, photos of me appeared in popular magazines like *Muscle & Fitness* and *Oxygen*. Not much longer after that, I was contacted by producers from the TV show *American Gladiators*, asking me to audition to be a gladiator. Ironically, I had been an American Gladiator for Halloween multiple times because I was obsessed with the show, just like every other kid born in the '80s. Somehow, among all of the professional athletes, stunt men, and longtime industry standouts, they chose me.

A haircut, some pink dye, and a tiny silver uniform, and "Phoenix" was born. The show will go down as one of my favorite experiences in my life, filled with great people and a greater understanding of the television business. I was very green, so in a way when the show was canceled it was the best thing for me. During that season I spent so much of my focus identifying myself for my external qualities and accolades, just like in college, that I never developed my own identity. With the show over I was lost and very unsure of where my life was going to go and, frankly, how I was going to pay for it. I didn't have a job and still was not using my college degree, so I threw myself into fitness modeling.

During this time, I moved to Los Angeles with the intent to truly find my purpose. Let me tell you, this was a struggle, especially since I was letting the outside world get in the way of building a healthy inside. Even though I was training and teaching fitness classes, I was living the opposite of a healthy life.

I was always in a good mood when I booked a modeling gig because I felt important and valuable, but in order to get ready for it I would have to crash-diet to prepare. With undereating a few weeks in advance and cutting major fluids, my obsession with how I looked and being "small enough" and "lean enough" was the only thing getting me through it.

Then after the photo shoot ended, I would binge all that night, usually with pizza, lots of sweets, and always some cocktails. These unhealthy habits began to turn into a huge problem for me because I started to have a very distorted image of myself. Even when I was in good shape, I still was never small enough. At each meal and in front of every mirror, I was tearing myself down.

At my lowest point, I remember binging, but through my education in the training field, I knew that if I threw up soon enough the calories would not have an impact on my body. The fact that that thought crossed my mind scared the shit out of me. All I could think was, "Am I really at the brink of an eating disorder? How could I let this go so far?"

This was a huge turning point for me, and instead of using exercise to mitigate my self-doubt, I began to use health and fitness as a way to mentally get healthy again. Rather than always judging myself, it was time to let myself "be human."

It's no surprise that over the next year my training business began to thrive. I was finally starting to put my best self forward, and people were responding to that. Through my own experience, my understanding of how to help people with much larger issues in their life dramatically grew, and I did it all through health and fitness.

This is what became my passion. My purpose. The momentum did not stop, and I started to get on the radar of prestigious wellness brands like *Men's Health* and *Women's Health, Muscle & Fitness*, and yes, *The Biggest Loser*.

On *The Biggest Loser* my approach is not one of tough love, though I set a tough standard: eat clean but highly nourishing foods, exercise right, and, most of all, learn to believe in and listen to yourself. All rules I live by. During my first two seasons on the show my team took home the prize, and that's exactly what I want for you—to finally win by overcoming the challenges of achieving your best body and healthiest life.

KEEPING IT REAL

If I'm being honest, I'm writing this book now because I spent many years confused about the role exercise and diet were supposed to have in my life. I made many of the same mistakes you're probably making right now. And even though I might have looked healthy on the outside, my mind-set created a dangerous relationship that made the way I was feeling unlivable.

Spending time in the gym or eating the right foods became a burden. I can't tell you how many times I wanted a dessert or the ability to take a day off, and my mind insisted, "You can't do this. That's not healthy! You'll get fat!"

The problem wasn't with my workouts or the meals I prepared. It was with me, my understanding of who I was, who I wanted to be, and what I could become. I finally embraced my personality and used it to build the foundation of the real me. Instead of condemning myself for how critical I was, I celebrated it by using it as an asset—daily checklists, brand-new Tupperware for all the meals I was prepping, and actually acknowledging my successes (even if they came in the form of a day with no negative self-talk) versus passing over them to beat myself up for some stray imperfect action that day.

Once I changed that perspective, I gave myself permission to be true to myself. I recognized the necessity of confidence, realizing I'm human (and fallible), and doing the best I can (which sometimes includes eating dessert and taking days off). That was when everything changed: in my life, in the lives of my friends and family and, maybe most important, in the lives of the people I train.

My secret: I learned to connect to the individual nature of what I needed. I looked at my personality, my traits, and all the pieces of the puzzle that make me *me*. I stopped the one-size-fits-all mentality that I had when it came to what I ate, when and how I worked out, and the lifestyle I was leading. And in turn, that shift allowed me to focus less on what everyone else was doing and more on what I needed—on my own goals and the way I could reach them. I began to create a routine of eating healthy and working out that made sense for me. As a result, I didn't just look good on the outside anymore, but I was happier, healthier, and more successful in all areas of my life.

If you're looking for a book on why you should follow the latest exercise trend or eat (or not eat) entire food groups to get thin fast, I won't waste your time with the same old message. Your frustration is real. And if you're like most people, you're probably tired of the endless diets and "get fit fast" promises that use and abuse your emotions and expectations. Or maybe you're simply looking for a change—something that doesn't just have to be a short-term fix, that works and then stops working.

This book is less about providing a "magic bullet" solution and more about simplifying what is most effective when it comes to nutrition and exercise, filtering out what doesn't matter and what doesn't work, and showing you how to finally be successful based on your personality and your specific needs. This is your solution, and one that can write a new story for your body. I'll help you understand why your previous attempts failed and what you can do to make sure that doesn't happen again.

These programs are the most effective methods I've come across in weight loss. I live my life based on what's in this book. Backed by science, tested and retested over the years, this plan will get your body to trust you again and shed weight fast because, just like you, it doesn't want to carry it anymore!

I'll teach you to believe in the power of your words and in yourself. Together, we will form a team that will bolster your strengths, navigate you through problem behaviors, and help you finally start living in a positive and vibrant way.

These are more than just words on a page. This is your blueprint, which means you have a choice: acknowledge that you need to consider your personality in any weight-loss program, and you will drop pounds and transform your life. Or you can continue to take shortcuts, ignore what will help you be successful, and continue to be frustrated by all the "general" diet and fitness information. The choice is yours, and I'm willing to take you on the journey if you commit to doing it with me.

have done the reps and work at ground zero every day with people who are fighting for their weight loss and better health, desperate to find a solution.

I don't want you to believe the lie that it's too hard to change your body. Every successful program starts with one common trait: you have to build an approach around the personality and preferences of each individual.

I cannot be successful with a client without doing this. If I said the same thing to five different people, in the same room, they would all perceive it a different way. This program is about understanding your unique personality traits and how to tap in to the diet and fitness regimen that will change your life once and for all. It's a revolutionary system based on the latest science of behavioral change.

If you've been looking for a fresh point of view that gives you the ability to navigate otherwise unseen potholes in your weight-loss journey, then you've made the right choice in picking up this book.

HOW TO USE THIS BOOK

My program is designed to activate you into this new way of living by using the qualities you already possess, so that you can experience remarkable change in just four weeks.

Let's walk through how that will happen: In Part 1, I'll introduce you to the program by sharing some key information about personality, how your body talks to you, and my foolproof ways that help your body burn fat. Together, we'll explore how ready you are, because readiness tremendously affects motivation by identifying what "stage of change" you are in—this is one of the more exciting parts of the journey! You'll also take a fun but critical twenty-question assessment to identify your dominant personality. Are you an "Organized Doer," "Swinger," "Rebel," "Everyday Hero," or "Never-Ever"?

In Part 2, now that you know your type, I'll give you a detailed diet that will be most effective for your personality, plus other important information you'll need for success, including meal plans, shopping lists, and recipes for the next four weeks.

Next, in Part 3, I'll get you moving with advice on how and when to work out, and I'll provide you with my effective and empowering 16-Minute Jen Bod Workouts. Finally, in Part 4, I'll help you complete your journey by giving you a maintenance plan and further tools and motivation that will serve you the rest of your life. Just because the book is at its end doesn't mean we are. This section is all about setting you up for the road ahead and reminding you that I'll always be there to be a part of your process.

Living at your best demands that you be honest with yourself—

your actions, your habits, your responses—and this is why it's critical that we'll delve so deeply into personality. It takes courage to own up to what isn't working for you and what you may need to change. This also includes understanding and celebrating who you are so you can be a part of a plan that actually works for you.

PART 1

DIET AND PERSONALITY

CHAPTER 1

YOUR PERSONALITY, YOUR PLAN

The biggest flaw I see in most diets is their one-size-fits-all approach. So many diets fail because they don't take into consideration individual tendencies or triggers, motivational patterns, or lifelong habits that are ingrained into our personalities. Even someone with the strongest willpower in the world can find it tough to stick to a plan that works for someone else but not for them. In truth, there's no diet that is perfect for all people. It's a matter of being a student of yourself, learning what is best for you, and putting your findings into action. I'm here to help you do that.

What makes my program unique is that it addresses the crucial issue most other diets ignore—the psychological and behavioral factors that make us all so different. From those factors, I have created nutrition plans tailor-made for each of you. I provide specific techniques to help each type of dieter on their journey and to spot common pitfalls they experience and navigate through them. My program will also give you a real insight into your personality—those characteristic patterns of motivation and behavior that define you—thus helping you get on a diet and exercise plan that you will not only stick to but thrive in.

To develop this program, I've used the information and insights gained over a decade of helping people lose weight and get in shape. Everyone's personality is unique, and what they need in the form of support and coaching is always very different. Customizing my role for each person is critical, and having very little time to do it is always a huge challenge. One week could mean success or failure for somebody. My clients look to me with complete trust. They count on me to guide them toward a thinner, more fit body—and that's what I'll be doing for you.

My program is infused with science. Many studies have been done in behavioral science over the years, but only recently has there been a growing research interest in the association of weight loss and gain with personality traits. If you've struggled with weight issues, fear not! It boils down largely to your diet personality—and science proves it! There is a lot more to dieting and weight control than just calorie counting, so drop the shame and the "I keep failing" attitude, and set yourself up for success!

Being overweight used to be such a clear science. If you were overweight, it meant you ate too much and exercised too little. End of story.

But hold on: if that were really the case, there'd be no need for me to write this book. It turns out that for the up to 60 percent of Americans who are overweight or obese, this explanation may be faulty and not the whole truth.

Recent breakthroughs have suggested that it's not just how much you eat or exercise that influences how you look and feel. The science of weight loss may be significantly linked to your psychological profile. Researchers have discovered that certain personality traits may determine, in large part, the type of diet approach you need to follow to lose weight and keep it off for the long haul.

This is less about labeling you as a certain "type" of person and more about understanding your own personality and how personality-specific strategies can help you finally drop the unwanted pounds and keep them off for good.

One of the leading theories suggests that personality traits can be grouped into five main categories: agreeableness, conscientiousness, extraversion, neuroticism, and openness. The five personality types in this book, as you'll see, are grounded in these findings. Each personality has many subtraits, of course. For example, trust is an aspect of agreeableness, and anxiety is an aspect of neuroticism. People can also be a combination of different types—something I agree with fully.

In several studies, researchers linked conscientiousness to better weight control, and I think there's a certain logic to this. Think about it: if you have a conscientious personality, you're probably more likely to develop good habits and less likely to engage in harmful behaviors. Conscientious people concentrate on specifics. They make daily plans and usually stick to them. They make to-do lists. All of these actions encourage positive and healthy behaviors.

By contrast, certain personality factors can make us prone to weight gain. Consider research from the National Institute of Aging that was published in 2011 in the *Journal of Personality and Social Psychology*, which looked at the connection between personality and weight control. According to this study, people who were impulsive were most likely to be overweight. In fact, study participants who scored high on impulsivity weighed an average of 22 pounds more than those at the lowest end of impulsivity.

And get this: those same researchers discovered that people who are impulsive—and disorganized—tend to have larger bellies and hips compared with individuals who are more imaginative, open to action, trusting, and modest.

It makes sense, if you think about it: those extra pounds can be a very physical reminder of the inability to control impulses, and people who repeatedly gain weight may start to perceive themselves to be, or to actually become, more impulsive and less disciplined.

And the list goes on and on. Researchers from the University of Washington in St. Louis found that people who score high in the personality trait of "novelty seeking" tend to be thrill seekers, become easily bored, and try to avoid monotony. Thus, they overeat to avoid boredom, and not surprisingly, their overeating contributes to weight gain. This study was published in the *International Journal of Obesity* in 2007.

So what's it all mean to you?

It should be a breath of fresh air—finally a plan designed for your body! You can't just up and change your personality. That's out of the question. The world needs you to be *you*, and I need you to celebrate that fact.

FIVE CORE PERSONALITY TYPES

After years working with hundreds of clients, I developed a unique weight-loss system grounded in research and shaped by my interaction with real people. It has become the backbone that allows for fast and long-lasting success for my clients (and myself!). It all began years and years ago at my first job in LA, when I was teaching boot camp classes at Pulse Fitness Studio. In the beginning, I was so focused on the programming, arranging the right music, and helping clients learn the movements that I did not initially see what has become the foundation of my training style: catering to individual personalities.

One day, as I was teaching a class, I noticed that only half of the class was responding positively to some of my motivational feedback. It seemed as if half of the class absorbed what I said, became even more engaged, and pushed harder on the workouts. Meanwhile, the other half was an odd mix of either disengaged and "busy" on their phones or indifferent to what I said and acting no better or worse than when we started.

What did this mean? Was I a bad coach? Was I annoying them? Was I talking too much? Or—as I eventually discovered—were my words not personal enough to reach all the personalities in the room?

As time went on, I found myself paying more attention to the different people in my classes and their traits. This hands-on experience is what helped me develop the five core personalities. And my ability to effectively communicate and help different people shaped my entire philosophy.

It became clear that I had to apply the principles not only during workouts, but also with nutrition, habits, and lifestyle decisions. As I worked with more people, I gained a better understanding of each personality type and the approach that worked best. My system became so foolproof because it wasn't just what I was having my clients do—it was *how* I was helping them take control and do it.

Many years later, I've identified five core personality types and the traits connected to each. Most important, I've learned that because each personality influences certain workout and diet preferences, there are personality-specific techniques for success (and preventing failure) that will simplify the process of building a healthier lifestyle.

The five core personality types are the following:

- **The Organized Doer**

- **The Swinger**

- **The Rebel**

- **The Everyday Hero**

- **The Never-Ever**

Everyone has a dominant type, and you'll determine which is yours by taking the assessment in Chapter 4. **The Organized Doer** is a type A personality who craves routine and rules, so that's exactly what they will receive because it drives their success! Checking off boxes is not stress inducing but rather meditative and an effective way to stay on track.

The Swinger is the adventurous type who follows the trendiest fads. Their success is rooted in a program that offers variety, change, and the ability to actively determine food and workout decisions each day.

The Rebel tends to be impulsive and noncommittal. They need to be given the opportunity to find their own flow in their day, and to be provided with flexible guidelines offering plenty of variety.

If you're an **Everyday Hero,** you probably always put yourself last and are happy to bend over backward for others. While this is admirable, it means you rarely accommodate yourself, even if you know it's necessary. The key for Everyday Heroes is building a plan that is streamlined and easy to set up, with as few obstacles as possible.

Finally, **the Never-Ever** is someone who's disconnected from their health and fitness or may have even given up. They require a plan that allows them to take a step back (and sometimes away from their negative self-talk) to get a macro view of their lives in order to open their minds to personal choices on a micro level. Their program is designed to help them break the vicious cycle and teach them how to be in control of the decisions that influence behavior.

Very soon, I'll help you understand your personality and what triggers you (in both a negative way and a positive way). This is invaluable because once you understand why you act and react the way you do to certain fitness and diet plans, then you can find the right approach for your style, meaning you're more likely to stick with the plan for everlasting health and weight loss.

Remember, dieting, fitness, and health are personal, and it is up to you to honor what is best for you. The reality is that there never will be any one person exactly like you. You are one-of-a-kind—a living, breathing bundle of beauty and strength. So let's start acting like it and adapt everything to you! Once you embrace this approach, that's when everything becomes easier and transformation is in your grasp.

THE BLIND SPOT

We are all familiar with mirrors, and—if you ask me—they tend to have too much persuasion in our lives when it comes to our self-worth. We believe that the reflection we see in them is of the utmost importance. And it's a problem. Because the mirror is just a snapshot. Just an outward reflection. It's a small piece of a much bigger story. A much deeper story. And what you can't see in the mirror is who you are beneath the reflection and why it's hard to overcome the mental hurdles that block your journey.

Recently, I started training a woman named Sharon. An affluent executive in her midforties, she told me,

> You know, Jen, I've got it all now: the car I want, a second home on the beach, and plenty of money to do as I please. But I'm unhappy, and these days I hate most everything about myself. When I look at myself in the mirror, I see a woman who is getting buried by her weight, and I'm starting to lose sight of ever coming out of this. I'm the heaviest I've ever been, and trying to fit into my clothes makes me

so upset. I am desperate to go out and meet someone, but I just can't bring myself to do it because I feel so bad about myself and the way I look.

Believe it or not, from a motivational standpoint, this client had arrived at an ideal place to initiate change. Behavioral scientists have shown in studies that people are *loss aversive*. That means, roughly speaking, that we are more miserable losing something than we are happy gaining the same thing, and that this dislike spurs us on to make needed changes in our lives.

A study published in 2015 in the prestigious *New England Journal of Medicine* found that smokers were more likely to quit if they enrolled in a smoking cessation program that involved the loss of money if they failed. Not wanting to lose their monetary deposit, they were able to complete the program and, voilà, quit smoking.

Likewise, Sharon no longer wanted to live with so many limitations and miss out on her life. After a few weeks, the power of this programming was evident. She shed eleven pounds, and lost 10½ inches all over her body, while adding close to four pounds of body-curving muscle. She was vivacious, positive, and shining with energy; she became a different person.

But, in fact, she was not anyone new. That woman had been there all along; she just needed help coming back to life. This is why the mirror is misleading. We can only see who we are in the present, not what lives within and not where we could be in a week . . . a month . . . a year . . . or even ten years. I challenge you to look through the mirror to see what lives within you, and see (like I do) that it's something incredible.

Does any of Sharon's process sound familiar? Are you having a "how did I end up here?" moment?

Ask yourself this next question, the most important question that you need to keep front and center going forward: "What am I not willing to lose out on anymore?"

Dating?
Travel?

Playing with your kids?

Feeling confident?

Self-pride?

Love?

Learning?

Health?

Wherever you are, own your position, but commit to moving forward. Take action and relieve yourself of how big or small that action is because my priority for you is progress, not perfection. Begin to consider how possible your progress is, as is your success. Take positive steps toward improving the way you see yourself. Think of your good points; acknowledge them and believe in them.

Also, do me a favor and put yourself first for a change! Step into your own purpose, be bold, and have an empowered heart and mind to start living healthfully. You are unique and individual, worthy of consideration and acceptance, especially from yourself. I don't know about you, but I want to be fit, capable, and connected well into my sixties, seventies, and eighties. Believe it or not, that decision begins now.

This Time Will Be Different (If You Follow This Advice)

Before we go any further, I want you to do me a favor. I want you to decide that you will take on not only the tasks that will change your body, but also those that will change your mind.

You just read about Sharon and her incredible success. While you will go through similar steps, the biggest difference in Sharon's journey this time (compared with her previous failures) is that she was able to change her mind-set *before* she started.

With this program you're going to see some incredible changes—and fast—but I care more about what happens beyond the weight loss. I don't want you to *ever* return to a frustrated state, whether it's five months or five years from now.

The one thing I want you to embrace during this program is the fact that we are all different. Love your personality type (which you'll soon learn more about), and ask yourself if you are living to your full capacity, or, as I call it, "living with your whole heart."

The day-to-day challenges of life can be difficult, and we often don't take the time to understand and process the effect they have on our health. For most people, these challenges are the constant questions and fears about who you are, what you can achieve, and how you can overcome hurdles and barriers. This fear distorts your sense of self to the point that it makes it harder to fully invest in certain goals you set. This can not only be controlling, but it also often masquerades as shame appearing in the form of negative self-talk, poor food choices, and avoiding new challenges.

You're probably most familiar with this process as it applies to exercise and nutrition plans and the constant doubt about whether you have what it takes to be successful on them. To overcome this vicious process, I want you to double down and invest in *you*. Embrace your uniqueness and pour your heart into loving who you are, not just *after* your transformation but *right now*.

Go into each day understanding that you're not perfect but with the knowledge and confidence that you are tapping in to who you are and applying that to who you want to become. This book is *not* about changing you. It's a call to adventure to honor the real you.

If you take this step, *everything* you read in this book will be more important, more powerful, and more effective. It will also help you actually enjoy the process.

CHAPTER 2

ARE YOU READY?

E very time I meet a new client, I begin with the same question: "Why are you here?" Usually, it is followed with answers such as, "I want to lose weight," "I want to improve my health," "I want to be able to play with my kids," "I want to look amazing in a bikini," and so forth.

These are the answers that most people give, but they are cursory responses. They do not reflect the mind-set that leads to long-term change. If you want fast results *and* results that last, we need to tap in to something much deeper. The first answer is great—and still important—but it leaves you with an incomplete puzzle. Once you learn how to fully understand your "why," that's when change becomes a habit and a lifestyle.

You see, there are two types of "whys": the why that comes from extrinsic motivation and the one that comes from intrinsic motivation. Extrinsic motivation is external. It stems from wanting to get in shape for a vacation, attend a high-school reunion and look fabulous, fit into a wedding dress or rock an attention-getting bathing suit, or attain other appearance-inspired goals.

Extrinsic motivation is often an effective motivator when you are getting started on a diet, but it can be fleeting as events pass and the results become temporary. If you rely solely on extrinsic motivation, it will be very difficult to possess the discipline needed from day to day, month to month, and year to year to maintain your new body.

Think about what I'm saying: what happens when the vacation is over, the reunion has ended, the wedding ceremony has passed, and it's no longer summer so who needs to fit into a bikini? I think you know the answer, because you've probably lived it. Extrinsic motivation is simply not enough to sustain a healthy (and hot) lifestyle.

Intrinsic motivation is different. It comes from within. It's the desire to be the healthiest you can be, for yourself and for your family. It is the desire to live longer and with a great quality of life. It is a willingness to prepare every day in order to maintain your full health potential while also experiencing your life at its fullest potential!

People exercise intrinsically, meaning they love what working out does to their state of mind, energy, and drive as much as how it changes their body. They are thriving on *feeling* strong versus just looking the part or following doctor's orders.

How can you get fired up to keep your weight off?

Right out of the gate, I need you to do some soul searching and establish baseline goals for yourself in order to resuscitate the "why" in your life: stamina to play with your kids and grandkids, climbing a simple flight of stairs without producing major huffs and puffs, improved heart health, greater energy, ability to concentrate, and a crowd favorite, extending your life.

Second, extrinsic motivation can turn into intrinsic motivation if you stick to your plan of healthy eating and exercise consistently over time. It did for me, so I know it can for you, too.

People who are successful in maintaining their weight have a sense of investment in themselves, they want to stay healthy for life experiences, and they're doing all the right things for genuinely deeper reasons. That's where I want you to be.

ARE YOU READY FOR CHANGE?

Very soon, you'll be starting your individualized and highly transformational diet. I've designed it so I'm there with you, every step of the way, as your personal coach. It's my duty to provide both sides of support: educating, guiding, and inspiring you to help you get where you want to be, but also sometimes dishing the tough-to-hear honesty that will help you through the moments where you question yourself.

If you follow the *Diet Right for Your Personality Type* plan, you will metabolize the fat off your waistline, hips, and thighs, and you will feel more connected to your body than ever before. Not only that, but you will also actually begin enjoying your food and your faith in the kitchen will be restored. No more second-guessing yourself on a meal-to-meal basis; you will know what behaviors affect your weight-loss success and be able to pilot each day with confidence. Most important, you will be able to free yourself of the guilt that has been connected to food and your weight.

In order for this transformation to work, you have to be prepared for the change ahead. The first step is determining if you're ready for change. People who want to break a bad habit—whether it's a poor diet, lack of exercise, smoking, or some other addiction—pass through a series of six predictable stages of change that help them modify those habits.

James Prochaska, PhD, professor of psychology at the University of Rhode Island, formulated this concept for people who wanted to conquer health-risky behaviors such as alcohol abuse and smoking. He reasoned that most people don't prepare themselves well enough for the big changes they want to make. As a result, they tend to fail again and again.

Prochaska termed his six stages the *transtheoretical model of behavior* or the *stages of change*. The stages range from being in total denial about the need to change all the way to permanent and positive lifestyle change. His model has gained widespread acceptance among psychologists and other health professionals, and its use is not limited to addiction. It is now being applied to diet and exercise.

In one study, researchers discovered that how well people do in a program directly correlates to the stage they are in before beginning it. For instance, researchers studied a worksite weight-loss program, in which a whopping 80 percent of the participants dropped out. They found that people who were either not ready to participate or merely toying with the idea of getting involved were the ones most likely to quit or fail to progress.

Experts agree that if you can identify and understand the importance of each stage and use specific strategies that are effective in each, you'll dramatically boost your chances of progressing from stage to stage and achieving your goals. Therefore, it only makes sense to help you become familiar with the six different stages. Pay close attention to the attributes so you can understand where you currently reside on the scale.

THE STAGES OF CHANGE

1. PRECONTEMPLATION

As you dip your hands into your daily bag of taco chips, you're thinking, "I need to give this up." But you're just not ready yet. . . . (But you will be soon, promise!) With excuses growing, today may not be that day. Or tomorrow, or the next day . . .

Please don't beat yourself up, because inaction doesn't necessarily mean failure. It may just mean you're not quite ready. You're in the precontemplation stage.

This means you may be in denial, or that you don't intend to change anytime soon. Or you just can't deal with your poor diet and fitness habits right now. You may even be in the dark about the benefits of a healthy diet or exercise, or believe that the benefits don't apply to you. Alternatively, you're fully aware of all the right reasons to get in shape, but you're simply not interested in doing it, or you haven't given too much thought to how to do it.

Deep down, you probably know that *not* making changes can lead to physical problems, including creeping obesity, diabetes, heart disease, high blood pressure, and many more health issues. A lot of people in this stage don't even want to read, talk, or think about these things.

STRATEGIES: Focus on your personal reasons for wanting to change—health, well-being, appearance, and more energy—and why an alteration in your diet and fitness level is important to you.

2. CONTEMPLATION

You're heading out for the night but everything you try on isn't zipping up or is too tight. You're discouraged, frustrated, and, if you're anything like me, starting to get emotional. As a result, you're seriously thinking about shedding pounds and opening up to a solution-oriented thought process. You're in what's called the contemplation stage—aware that you need to lose weight by having a more active role in your food choices and activity level. You're seriously considering it. But you haven't quite taken the plunge to take action yet.

Some personality types in this stage weigh the pros and cons of changing their behavior. Others are wishy-washy about doing it. Many types get stuck here because they've substituted the actionable benchmark that will have an impact on their weight loss for the mere thought of it. If this sounds like you, you're procrastinating.

Then there is the type who may feel pessimistic about changing their fitness habits: Can I stick to yet another diet? Will I fail? Do I have time to exercise? Will I even get results? How long is it going to take?

When I have clients contemplating change, I challenge them by having them identify their personal reasons to diet and exercise. In addition, I address with them what they are no longer willing to lose out on by *not* making any change.

Remember what I shared earlier? We are less inspired to make changes for what we could gain than we are when we are in jeopardy of losing something. I also help my clients knock down the barriers that block them from being more active, such as the ever-popular "not enough time to exercise." For example, I tell them to replace defeating self-talk like "Exercise takes too much time" with a positive approach: "Only twenty minutes of being active right now will make me feel better for the rest of the day in *every* way."

STRATEGIES: Envision yourself having lost the weight you want and being in better shape. See yourself wearing your two-piece or skinny jeans again. Focus on the disadvantages of being overweight and the advantages of being strong, lean, and fit (say, better health, so you can be a good role model for your kids). Be aware that within this stage, defeating self-talk may surface, so be prepared to meet it head-on with your passion, and give your goals a voice louder than the doubt.

If you're in the contemplation stage and want to move forward, think about why (or how) you gained the weight and got out of shape in the first place. List those reasons (such as stress, wrong diet, crappy nutritional habits, poor time management, emotional fatigue, etc.). Analyze the relationship you have with food and eating. Include the environment of where, when, and why you usually eat and sometimes overindulge: in your car; while watching TV; when you're depressed, bored, or stressed; while socializing; and so forth.

Spend time here. Assess these issues and give yourself honest feedback. Doing this will prepare you for the next stage. Before you move on, however, there's just one important point about the contemplation stage you should know: don't assume you're ready to lose weight because of pressure you feel from friends, family, the media, and society. You're at the brink of taking action, but the desire and motivation to change has to come from within you.

3. PREPARATION

Congratulations! You are anticipating your action stage and setting yourself up for success in the process. You've gotten rid of junk food from your pantry and fridge. You've looked at your weekly schedule and allotted time for workouts. You're in a positive headspace—turned down the volume on doubts and fears—and feeling empowered to succeed. You may have even set goals already and let your family and friends in on your plan. In short, you're feeling ready for commitment and are taking the right steps to begin.

STRATEGIES: Set a date for your first workout. Buy groceries for the first week of your diet. Tell your close friends, spouse, and co-workers that you plan to lose weight (going public will create a positive forum for accountability and make it harder to back out). Begin to see the freedom in following a diet that has you as the center of its focus.

4. ACTION

Welcome to the action stage.

You're *doing* it. You're changing your behavior. You're fully immersed in the weight-loss process, and you're following through with your personally tailored plan. Your cravings are tapering off, and positive feelings are beginning to reach into areas of your day that you didn't anticipate. The phrase "What took me so long?" continues to

The Rewards of Change

For you to progress from precontemplation to action and then to the final stages of change, the pros of changing your behavior must outweigh the cons. What lights you up? You will be an advocate only for the benefits of getting in shape that are of value to you. Here's a list of potential benefits I made. Which ones resonate with you? Can you add to this list? Invest a little time and really think about what motivates you.

- More attractive appearance
- Looking and feeling younger
- Strength
- Endurance
- Flexibility
- Higher metabolism
- Consistent weight control
- Prevention of bone and muscle loss
- Elevated energy
- Healthier heart, lungs, and circulatory system
- Prevention of serious hereditary diseases such as diabetes, certain cancers, heart disease, and stroke
- Injury prevention and/ or recovery
- Self-esteem
- Self-mastery, with renewed discipline and patience
- Stronger follow-through
- Owning your vulnerability
- Courage to get off the sidelines
- Improved memory
- Alertness and clearer thinking
- Better sleep
- Less depression
- Stress relief
- Better posture and body alignment
- Confidence
- Productivity at work
- Finding your voice
- Greater enjoyment of life
- Rejuvenation of your spirit

surface, and you, for the first time, maybe ever, are realizing the reason I wrote this book in the first place: because just as I believe, you are beginning to believe it, too . . . that you *can* do this!

STRATEGIES: Be vocal about your plan and goal. Accountability is one of the top factors in weight management. Include important people in your life so that you can access their support.

I want you to develop some adherence strategies. No matter what your personality type, there are behaviors you may default to when triggered. For example, if you're used to eating dessert after dinner, how can you prepare yourself to not default? Get rid of the sweets in your house and stop stocking your kitchen with high-calorie junk foods? Decide to have fresh fruit for dessert instead of cheesecake? Head to the gym to get your mind off that cheesecake?

Researchers call these strategies *lifestyle interventions*, which help counter your default, out-of-control eating. A number of years back, the American Heart Association (AHA) published a report in the journal *Circulation* that gave behavioral-health strategies to help people follow healthier lifestyles. Most were common-sense steps— things as simple as honestly writing down how much you exercise and what you eat each day and setting realistic goals for change.

My program of individually tailored diets is a good example of a lifestyle intervention, and one that is proven to work. A 2011 study in the *European Journal of Nutrition* found that when dieters are given a tailored eating plan of healthy food choices, they are more successful over the long term than they'd otherwise be on a fixed, cookie-cutter type diet. These dieters lost weight steadily over ten months, kept it off—and successfully changed poor eating habits.

When in the preparation stage, you want to have a structure and a plan. This could look something like this:

Every Sunday, look at your calendar and schedule your workouts for the next week, writing down potential obstacles and strategies for dealing with each of them. Track your progress. A journal or diary is one of the best tools for helping you stay focused (though not all personality types are successful with this). Ask friends and family for support. Consider enrolling in a class or program. Add variety. Keep things interesting by adding new activities or expanding your goals to make them more challenging.

Once you've leveled up your connection to these lifestyle changes, you'll drastically reduce your chances of reverting back to habits that don't serve you or your end goal.

JEN JUJU: Goal-Setting Secrets

We all need long-term fitness goals. Some examples: muscle and strength gains, a faster 5K time, competing in your first triathlon, surviving a spinning or CrossFit class, going on a hike without having to sit down every ten minutes to rest, and losing some weight.

I call these big-picture goals, and they're an important part of my whole coaching style and philosophy. Everyone should set them, and the preparation stage is a good time to do it.

How do you achieve your big-picture goals? Answer: baby steps. These are the day-to-day actionable activities you do to make your goals. Examples: eating a green veggie every day; beginning every day with a glass of water; working out twice a week, then peppering in more workouts as the weeks go by; practicing positive self-talk; and more. These keep you "in it." Plus, they give you feelings of accomplishment, measurable and tangible shifts in healthy behavior, and empowerment that comes with completing something you never thought you could—you know, daily game changers!

Start small and build. Begin to honor every accomplishment, no matter how small (a workout, a healthy meal, a walk around the block, etc.). The moment you look at what you can do versus what you couldn't do, everything will change for you.

5. MAINTENANCE

This is your victory lap! This is your time to celebrate success: you made it!

Maintenance means you've hit your ideal weight and want to keep it forever.

You'll launch into the process of sustaining positive changes in your lifestyle. You'll even sidestep temptations that may encourage relapse. Once in this stage, you're dedicated, and fitness has become a habitual part of your life versus part of a to-do list. You'll feel confident that you can carry out and protect your efforts of transformation.

Even the well-known National Weight Control Registry (NWCR) agrees. This organization was established in 1994 to observe and identify the characteristics of individuals who experienced successful long-term weight loss, defined as a loss of thirty pounds or more for one year or longer. In 2015, the organization concluded: "There is not a 'one size fits all strategy' for successful weight loss maintenance and that weight loss maintenance may require the use of more strategies by some individuals than others."

That is exactly what my experience has shown me, too: you need to adjust the keep-it-off strategies and tools for different personality types. What works for your best friend in keeping weight off may not necessarily work for you. Just as taking weight off requires a customized approach, so does keeping it off.

6. TERMINATION

This final stage is the pinnacle, honey! The top of Everest, the no-turning-back stage. You're different, better, awesome, and fantastic— inside and out. I am psyched for you, and you are now part of the most recent graduating class of Team Jen.

Imagine it: your healthy lifestyle is so much a part of you that you have zero compulsion to slip back into any weight-gaining behavior. For example, there is no way you'll go back to your sedentary lifestyle, no matter what. You're living life as if you never acquired bad habits in the first place. Staying fit and active now defines you.

When my clients reach this stage, I know that they can manage themselves spectacularly and even continue to make greater progress on their own. This is what I want for you, and I will get you there.

MOVING THROUGH THE STAGES

How you go through those stages is influenced by personality—which is why knowing your personality type will help you understand why certain challenges in life come easily, and others involve more of a struggle.

Let's say your personality is perfection-focused, analytical, and serious. You get immersed in the journey of thinking, researching, and analyzing—often for a long time—before you commit to starting a diet or joining a certain gym. Or maybe you're more of a spontaneous, adventuresome type who jumps into change fast and with both feet. Or you might be someone who puts others' needs ahead of your own—that's why you often lack the readiness to change your behavior. You may selectively attend to some things and not to others. The bottom line is that your inherent personality type indicates how you move through the various stages of change.

Evolving from one stage to the next, without skipping past any, is the key to your success. *You have to be honest about where you are.*

If you don't understand where you are and you try to jump into the action stage while still in the contemplation stage, then the process simply will not work. If you jump in halfheartedly, this will become the basis of your failure, but keep in mind that this is *not* reflective of your own abilities to ever achieve success here. Understanding this distinction is critical. Typically, I see people move on from one stage to another when they feel some level of discomfort in their daily lives—something as simple as being out of breath while going up stairs, not feeling attractive in clothes, or having a life-threatening weight-related condition such as an array of symptoms for heart disease. All of these events can spur people to want to change and have them charging into action without fully contemplating the steps necessary to modify their behavior to achieve their goal.

Keep in mind that your road to success will not be linear and that a break in resolution or even a relapse does not mean you have failed. These experiences texture your journey and are a chance to be a student of yourself. Your broken resolution doesn't mean that you aren't changing, but that you are learning and putting that information to use going forward. This is all part of the transformation process, so embrace it with clarity and self-love.

If you take away anything from this chapter, it should be that change is a process. Change does not have to be overly challenging, but it's also not a simple, single event. Accept this . . . and you can do the things necessary to move you through the stages of change.

CHAPTER 3

EAT RIGHT NO MATTER YOUR PERSONALITY TYPE

O f all the information out there on "healthy" and "effective" nutritional guidelines, it's easy to feel lost in the shuffle and overwhelmed with what to follow or believe. So many programs focus on opposite and extreme sides of the nutritional spectrum, creating confusion that becomes a roadblock for your willingness to even begin your diet.

This chapter will be different. It will be your mini life guide for food, equipping you with fundamental information and meal benchmarks based on optimal nutritional quality, timing, and portions. No matter what your personality, my staples of daily living for staying lean and connecting to your health apply to us all.

My nutritional philosophy is built on principles of properly fueling and nourishing your body. Even though you'll be following your own special diet, I will have you apply key strategies to maximize your success rate. Using these strategies, you will overcome an onslaught of major hurdles—junk food cravings, slow metabolism, bad food habits, and more—to stay fit for life. No more "good" diet days, "bad" diet days, or good me/bad me ... just some Jen-sense basics that will make your individualized diet work even better. Let's dig in.

BE A CONSCIOUS EATER

Awareness is the key to your weight-loss success. When it comes to each meal, practice *mindful* eating. In layman's terms, that means don't check out while you chow! I can't tell you how many times I've sat down for a meal, begun to eat, gotten caught up in conversation, and then looked down at my plate and thought, "Who ate all my food?" Confession: me!

I ate unconsciously for most of my life. I'd be so consumed with the next bite that I wouldn't even really notice the one I was chewing. I just mindlessly stuffed my face. Good food. Bad food. ALL food.

I want to point out that I wasn't consciously doing anything wrong, and neither are you! This habit stems from our increasingly fast-paced lives. We often show up at a meal starving because we were too busy and waited too long to eat. Many of us were also brought up from childhood to "finish what's on your plate!" None of this means you're doing anything wrong, but you should have an internal awareness of what you are doing so you don't automatically slip into ingrained bad habits at meals. This awareness will keep you in the driver's seat every time you sit down to eat.

Additionally, I want you to use your meals as opportunities to slow down for a moment during your day. Even a simple bowl of oatmeal at breakfast or a veggie wrap for lunch at your desk can provide a respite and an opportunity to unplug. Place your silverware or food down between bites, look up from your plate, taste—chew—breathe.

Let's also make an intention to eat more slowly. When you slow down, you eat less and give your body the time it needs to respond and tell you it's full. It helps digestion, and you'll have fewer cravings throughout the day. Being more mindful allows you to experience your food.

Close the book, shut off the television, put down your phone, and focus on your meal. See, savor, and sense your food as a gift and let its energy nourish your entire self. You may smile as you read this, maybe because it sounds a little corny, but I promise you—the difference in how you feel will be undeniable.

EAT "ONE-INGREDIENT" FOODS

A big key to losing weight and building lean muscle is a healthy metabolism—the process that turns food into fuel. One of the best ways to stoke metabolism is to eat what are called "one-ingredient foods."

What is a one-ingredient food, you ask? Exactly what it sounds like: a food with a single ingredient. Take a sweet potato, salmon, or a blueberry, for example. These foods have only one name to describe them. Nothing added; they're just what they are. You get the idea!

Compare such foods with processed foods you find in packages. They're full of many ingredients, most of which you can't even pronounce. Frankly, if you can't say 'em, don't eat 'em. Staying away from these foods is another key strategy for your success, because your body doesn't like them, recognize them, or even digest them properly—so often they convert to stored energy, accumulating as fat tissue.

Sometimes, even seemingly "healthy" foods like protein bars or canned shakes are highly processed and filled with low-quality ingredients. I'm not completely against these foods, as I would take them over what you usually get at any drive-through, but I do consider them a last-resort option.

One-ingredient foods are my first choice when it comes to what I put on my plate and are what I eat off that plate before anything else. They are priority foods, and I want you to look at them like that. These foods are easily recognizable *and* digestible in your body. This is critical when it comes to absorbing all the nutritional value of your meals but also for completing that exchange of unwanted pounds for lean muscle tissue. Not only that, but when you're doing this on a regular basis it affects your energy in your workouts, allowing you to max out the return on that investment of time and energy as well. Win-win!

In becoming more comfortable with this concept, get acquainted with the nutrition facts of the foods already in your home. By law, every ingredient must be listed, so read up on what you've been ingesting. If there is a long ingredient list or if there are items there that you don't recognize and can't pronounce, then I urge you to swap out those foods for others with as few ingredients as possible. A good rule of thumb is to keep as many one-ingredient foods on your plate at each meal as possible.

A Fatty Trifecta

If you want to keep those lost pounds off—and I mean forever—you've got to break up with three substances:

ADDED SUGAR

Added sugar means sugar added to foods: white sugar, brown sugar, high-fructose corn syrup, corn syrup, glucose, fructose, sucrose—really anything with *-ose* connected to the last syllable of the word. All that sweet crap can *and will* make you fat and, in turn, put you at risk for heart disease, diabetes, and other terrible health problems linked with being overweight.

LIQUID CALORIES

Liquid calories pack on more weight than normally fattening solid foods, a new study suggests. I'm talking about soft drinks or soda, booze, fruit drinks, fruit punch, and high-calorie beverages sweetened with sugar or high-fructose corn syrup (which, by the way, is more easily converted to fat than other sugars are).

Researchers analyzed the relationship between beverage consumption and weight gain among 810 adults and found that they started losing weight when they cut back on their liquid calories. So just because you're in maintenance mode doesn't mean you can go back to downing these empty calories. Stick with my hydration schedule and water-drinking guidelines; they'll keep you at your ideal weight.

SHELF-STABLE FOODS

Shelf-stable foods are those that can be safely stored at room temperature, or "on the shelf." These nonperishable products include canned and bottled foods, cookies (the fat-free kind, too, because they are loaded with sugar to compensate for the bad taste that comes with the lack of fat), chips, crackers, and processed foods in packages that do not require refrigeration until after opening. Shelf-stable foods are generally treated with heat and/or dried to get rid of food-borne germs that can cause illness or spoilage and are packaged in sterile, airtight containers. That's all fine and good, but shelf-stable foods tend to be low in nutrients and therefore not conducive to weight loss, weight maintenance, or good health. Stick to real one-ingredient foods (fresh produce, for example), and you'll maintain your weight without going out of bounds into this packaged nonsense.

EAT FAT-BURNING FUEL COMBINATIONS

The body works on two fuel tanks: carbohydrate/protein and fat/protein. Protein's primary function is to rebuild and repair your body, but it is also very good at making your metabolism work—which means more calories burned and a slim and smiling you. Your body *needs* to be challenged like this throughout the day to keep your body fat down, so keeping protein in most of your meals is key.

Foods high in protein rev up your metabolism, and that means your body gets good at burning fat and building lean muscle. Judging from the science, protein is definitely a fat-burner. In a study published in the *Journal of the Academy of Nutrition and Dietetics*, researchers demonstrated that higher-protein meals had a powerful fat-burning impact on overweight people, who are less efficient at metabolizing fat. The reason for protein's influence? It has a higher *thermic effect of food* (TEF) than carbs. This means that the body expends more energy to digest and absorb protein than carbohydrates. That energy comes from stored fat that is broken down and metabolized so it can be used for fuel. The net effect is more pounds burned off.

Other studies show that bumping up your dietary protein regulates your appetite better and tapers sugar cravings. Protein-packed foods supply amino acids, which are vital for metabolism and weight loss.

The absolute best protein in my book is fish. Why? Because it breaks down the fastest; its component amino acids get into your system quickly to start creating attractive muscle. The healthiest (and the tastiest, in my opinion) fish that I lean toward is salmon. It's loaded with omega-3 fatty acids, which help the body burn fat as well as improve skin, hair, joints, and heart health, while acting as a major anti-inflammatory agent for your whole body.

Now, understanding how fat and carbohydrates interact and what they do for you is just as important as adding protein if you want to get lean fast. Both protein and carbs are responsible for fueling and energizing your body, but the tricky part is that your body works from only one of these fuel tanks at a time. Put simply, when it comes to carbs and fat, you can eat *both* . . . just not at the same time. Let me dig in a little further here.

When you give your body both carbs and fat at the same time, it's going to decide which one to use and which one to store. For instance, when you eat peanut butter on toast, your body will go for the toast to break down and use first because carbohydrates are the body's primary source of energy. The peanut butter, then, which is very high in fat, digests much more slowly and is held to the side and stored. This is not good when what you're trying to train your body to do is use and burn off fat, NOT store it!

A similar example is the very popular avocado toast. This is one of the worst things you can order if you're trying to lose weight because of the carb and fat combination. If you're at your goal weight, you have more freedom to have the avocado toast, but if you want to *stay* at your goal weight I wouldn't take part in that too often. Buzzkill, I know.

The solution is this: fats are important to keep in your diet, so when you do have fats in your meal, make sure you don't have any carbohydrates with them. This puts your body in the position where it *has* to choose the fat to burn.

To take this a step further, a ton of science supports the reduction, if not elimination, of carbohydrates later in your day and the prioritizing of fats, protein, and vegetables instead. When you ease back on carbs, your body's blood sugar levels fall a bit, causing the pancreas to manufacture less insulin. With less insulin to draw on, the body is forced to burn stored fat for fuel, resulting in weight loss.

In addition, you'll be relying more on fat than carbs for fuel, so your fat will begin to mobilize instead of accumulate, and your weight will drop again.

Your starting lineup for healthful fats includes olive oil, coconut oil, avocados, nuts, and seeds. These supply essential fatty acids (EFAs), which are healthy fats that we need for many different processes in the body. EFAs increase the production of fat-burning enzymes, catalysts that ignite fat burn.

Energy Density: The Key to Feeling Full

Would you like to feel more full but without adding extra calories? Then choose foods with a low energy density. Energy density (ED) is defined as the number of calories in a given food divided by the number of grams in a serving.

You can check the Nutrition Facts label of packaged foods to calculate the ED. Take a slice of wheat bread, for example. To figure out its ED, divide the calories per serving by the weight of the serving in grams. For bread, the equation is 78 calories divided by 28 grams = an approximate ED of 3.

Foods can have an energy density ranging from 0 to 9 calories per gram. Higher-fat foods tend to fall closer to 9 calories per gram (high energy density), while foods with lots of fiber and water, such as veggies, fruits, soups, and salads, contain far fewer calories per gram (low energy density). When you swap out high-energy-density foods with low-energy-density ones, you feel full longer, thanks to the combination of high protein, fiber, and water content.

Here's how you can use some simple math to figure out whether the ED in the food you're eating is high, medium, or low:

ED below 0.6	Very low	Most fruits and vegetables, reduced-fat milk, light yogurt, and broth-based soups
ED 0.6 to < 1.5	Low	Flavored reduced-fat yogurt, cottage cheese, low-fat meats such as skinless poultry and pork tenderloin; many breakfast cereals, eaten with low-fat or fat-free milk; eggs; corn; legumes; pasta; rice
ED 1.5 to < 4.0	Medium	Dried fruit, breads, some snack foods, hard cheeses, salad dressings, higher-fat meats
ED 4.0 < 9.0	High	Crackers, most chips, chocolate, candy, cookies, nuts, bacon, butter, oil

Source: D. A. Hammock, "Lose Weight—Without Going Hungry," *Good Housekeeping*, 2004.

High-ED foods don't create any kind of satiety—they contain no fiber and no quality ingredients that really feed your body. You have to be thoughtful about where you get your calories.

AVOID PORTION DISTORTION

Now, in no way do I want you to obsess over portions, but I can't have you disconnect from them, either. It is critical for you to have an honest connection (which goes back to our discussion on mindfulness earlier) with your food and, most notably, how much of each food group you're consuming. Although it can be tough to gauge how much is too much, focusing on food-to-plate ratios is an easy technique that will offer you accountability on your plate. Use your plate as a pie chart: roughly 70 percent of the food should be grown from the earth—vegetables, fruits, or seeds—and 30 percent can be from an animal source—dairy, meat, or fish.

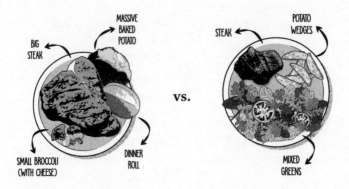

Some people are going to need a little more food than others. Here's a trick I share with my clients: portion your plate appropriately, sit down, and eat your meal while periodically putting your silverware down in between bites. Once the food is gone, you're done . . . BUT, if in an hour, you're like, "Whoa, I'm ravenous, I need to eat more," well, then, that's okay! You're allowed to eat a bit more, but nine times out of ten you'll find that you're not hungry.

Lightbulb moment: Give yourself a little time to digest, and you'll realize that your first-plate portions are enough to nourish your body, and your days of overeating will come to an end.

So with portions, you can simplify serving-size questions by loading your plate with as many one-ingredient foods as you can: brightly colored squash or sweet potatoes, deep green cruciferous and leafy vegetables, and a flaky whitefish or other lean protein flavored with lemon and herbs. This is what you need in order for your muscle tissue and energy to be supported, as well as for your metabolic furnace to stay in play.

Eat this way consistently. *Consistency* is necessary in getting the body you want and maintaining it.

More on Portions

These programs are built for an average woman, 5'3" to 5'7", with the goal of weight loss. If you are a man, increase the portions in each recipe by 30 percent.

FIGHT FAT WITH FIBER

One of the least-honored nutrients in our diets is fiber, a crucial component of any fat-burning meal plan and found mainly in fruits, vegetables, nuts, seeds, and grains. Besides making you feel full, fiber also speeds food through your digestive tract.

Need to trim off belly pudge? Fiber to the rescue. A study published in the journal *Obesity* reported that for every 10-gram increase in soluble fiber people ate over a period of five years, they had nearly a 4 percent reduction in deposits of *visceral fat*, a type of fat that pads your stomach and other internal organs. It is associated with serious health problems, including type 2 diabetes.

Found in oats, beans, and some fruits and veggies, soluble fiber is soluble in water, which means that it breaks down to form a gel. Another type of fiber in foods is insoluble fiber, found mostly in whole grains. It passes through the body virtually unchanged and helps maintain a healthy digestive tract by speeding up the passage of food and waste.

Sufficient intake of both types of fiber has also been linked to a lower risk of heart disease and several forms of cancer. Fiber also reduces the risk of digestive troubles, such as hemorrhoids, diverticulitis, and ulcers.

For fiber to work its magic, everyone needs about 20 to 35 grams of it a day. Making that quota is not all that difficult. Simply gravitate toward one-ingredient foods and keep your distance from anything highly processed. If you feel that your diet lacks this key nutrient, or you want to fight fat with fiber, start by eating more of the following "fiber all-stars."

FIBER ALL-STARS

Beans and lentils
Flaxseed
Chia seeds
Oats
Quinoa
Spinach
Almonds
Squash
Cruciferous vegetables (cauliflower, broccoli, Brussels sprouts, or cabbage)
Sweet potatoes
Pears
Avocados
Split peas
Artichokes

TIME YOUR MEALS AND WORKOUTS

People frequently ask me whether it's a good idea to work out on an empty stomach. This is a personal decision, but I always do. When you put food in your body and try to train, your system pulls blood from your extremities to focus on the digestion of the food in your stomach—a feeling I don't like when I'm training because it limits my productivity. Additionally, I want my body burning off the sugar store that's already in my body, and not what I've just put in my stomach.

I would advise eating immediately after a workout, so your body can begin the process of replenishing, restoring, and rebuilding. The best refueling meal includes lean protein, along with a one-ingredient carb, such as a sweet potato, or even a smoothie made with protein powder, fruit, and some raw oats.

For all my vegans and vegetarians out there, here is a list of my favorite proteins that you can sub in for any of the proteins I have listed in the recipes. Aim for variety but be more inclusive of the ones your body responds to the best:

- 2 to 3 tablespoons algae (chlorella/spirulina)
- 1½ cups artichokes
- 1 cup black-eyed peas
- 1½ cups green peas
- 1 cup edamame
- 1 cup tempeh
- 1 cup tofu
- ¾ cup lentils
- ¾ cup black beans
- 3 tablespoons hemp seeds
- ½ cup pumpkin seeds
- 2 cups spinach

HYDRATE RIGHT

Water covers more than half the earth, makes up most of our body weight, and is the most essential nutrient for life. Yet it is still little more than a nutritional footnote. Most of us don't drink nearly enough of it.

You've probably been told to drink at least 8 cups of pure water a day. Well, that may not be enough. You require between eight to ten and a half 8-ounce glasses of water a day just to support the basic functions of life. Yet a normal, healthy adult pees out almost 6 cups of water a day. And that doesn't take into consideration fluid losses from daily activity, workouts, or a hot day under the sun. Are you starting to see what I see? You definitely need more water!

The more water my clients drink, the more efficiently they drop pounds, and it will be the same for you. Water is such a huge influential factor in losing weight that if you literally changed nothing else in your lifestyle but drank your daily minimum amount of water, you would likely lose weight. One study reported that drinking 2 cups of water increased calorie burning by 24 percent for up to an hour after ingestion. In another study, drinking that same amount of water bumped up metabolic rate by 30 percent within ten minutes.

On each plan, I'll have you drinking a lot of water throughout the day. By week four, you'll be drinking 75 ounces of water or more each day. You will learn how to ramp up your hydration gradually, from week to week, and as you do, you'll enjoy watching your body let go of all the weight that's been holding you back from your goal.

No matter where you are or what you're doing, keep these strategies in your back pocket to draw on. Use them as a template to navigate meals, trips, parties, and even just difficult days. When you do, that is when you begin to build momentum on your weight-loss journey. I need you to prove to yourself that you can get through those tough moments and make a better decision than you would have before you were willing to bet on yourself and believe you could really do this. These strategies will help you amplify the individual diet plan I give you and have you living without limits for the first time in your adult life. It is no longer about what you would like to eat—it's about choosing something you want even more: to lose weight and get in the best shape of your life.

CHAPTER 4

WHAT'S YOUR PERSONALITY TYPE?

Maybe you've always thought of yourself as an extrovert—you know, the high-fivin' go-getter who can crash any party and fit right in; or maybe you are more of the introvert who recharges by eliminating stimulation and finds comfort in routine.

But when it comes down to the important business of dieting to get healthy and in shape, over the long term, you need a broader, more in-depth insight into your personality so that you can follow a program that suits you best. Now you may not know this, but when it comes to dieting, you have specific patterns that stem from your personality type.

Drumroll, please: Personality matters. *You matter.* If personalities weren't important, introverts would be jumping up to give toasts and extroverts wouldn't mind keeping quiet. The same is true for diet. And while this topic may have gotten lip service before, no one has truly looked at you: your soul, your heart, what motivates you, and what keeps you from making the most important changes in your life.

When the wrong diet is paired with the wrong personality, it's a matchmaking nightmare because you feel disconnected from the plan, so your motivation and ability to succeed go out the window. While a prescribed and structured meal plan may appeal to one person, having the freedom to plan meals would inspire another.

Jumping into a diet without any sense of who you are and what issues you may want to address is just not the best way to proceed. So rather than keep diet-hopping to hope you find the one that matches you, why not put yourself under the microscope for a minute and give yourself the attention you deserve to win. You've got to reconnect with yourself and what motivates you in order to succeed. What are your tendencies, traits, and triggers? What piques your curiosity? What makes you feel hopeful? What makes you feel understood? What triggers hopelessness or the daunting feeling that this will all be for naught—again? What obstacles always get in your way of establishing a positive rhythm when it comes to your health?

Remember, I take a deeper look into the person and not just into the programming to see what success is for you: the stuff your average dietitian would consider irrelevant, including basic chitchat that reveals golden nuggets of information about the real you—the you that is brave, that stays positive in the face of adversity, and that has moments of vulnerability and imperfection.

If you match your personality with your way of eating, you will lose the weight and keep it off. I know it because I've lived it alongside my clients over and over again. I've found that people who take time to determine their diet personality type and follow diets that nurture that type are more likely to be successful in losing weight and keeping it off. So any sound nutritional plan needs to start with an honest look at your default reactions and style of eating. The assessment I've developed will give you that reality check and start you on the right road, finally.

I cannot wait for you to take this revealing assessment. It will define your personality while showing you how to embrace it, and *this* is the first step toward dieting success. Once you've finished the assessment, it will reveal which of the five diet personality types you have. From here you'll be ready to jump into the next chapters, where you'll find a diet program that I have designed just for your type. That means you'll have a customized approach that will make it easier for you to start burning fat efficiently, get to your weight goal quickly—and stay there.

THE PERSONALITY ASSESSMENT: WHAT TYPE OF DIETER ARE YOU?

Read through each of the following statements and responses carefully. Circle just ONE response per question—the honest response that best describes you.

1. **When there's good news and bad news, which one do you want to hear first?**

   a. Just give me the facts; I'll decide whether it's "good" or "bad."

   b. Start with the good! Whatever the bad is, it will be manageable.

   c. I'm indifferent about the order, just don't leave out any of the juicy details.

   d. Bad, let's get it out of the way.

   e. I can never answer this question because it changes based on my mood and who I'm talking to.

2. **What builds interest for you in getting involved in a fitness or nutrition program?**

   a. I like to see the results of my efforts and experience an "I did that!" feeling of accomplishment.

   b. It's fun to get in the whirlwind of a project but ideally without the pressure of having a deadline to complete it.

   c. It's a great way to meet people—I'm always more invested when I'm accountable to a team or community.

   d. When I know my involvement may benefit others, I like to step up, plus it always makes me feel good about myself.

   e. It's an opportunity to tap in to new things I haven't tried and keeps my big-picture hope of reaching my goals alive.

3. **Of the following, what throws you off the most and/or is your biggest pet peeve?**

   a. Lateness or tardiness in others.

   b. Feeling restricted by too many rules and/or feeling obligated to do something.

   c. Boredom.

   d. Overscheduling myself and running out of time.

   e. Outside opinions. Don't tell me what to do.

4. **How do you feel about leftovers or doggy bags?**

   a. I transfer any leftovers to their own container at home and store them. I'll eat just a few bites or nothing at all.

   b. I pack them up and eat them on the way home or later that night. The end of one meal is often the start of my next!

   c. I don't really like leftovers. It's boring to eat the same food two or more days in a row.

   d. I love 'em because I can repurpose leftovers for tomorrow's meals.

   e. I may never eat them, but I always feel better when I keep them.

5. **If someone tells an embarrassing story about you, how do you react?**

   a. I become shy and embarrassed for a short period of time.

   b. LOL, what? I did that?

   c. I jump in and tell what *really* happened in the story.

   d. I laugh along, while adding in self-deprecating remarks.

   e. I smirk while the person blabs on, thinking, "Well, look who's throwing the first stone."

6. **If you found twenty dollars, what would you do?**

   a. I'd put it toward a bill.

   b. I'd tuck it in a safe place, probably forget about it, and then redis-cover it a month later.

   c. Woo-hoo, let's spend it! Coffee, anyone?

   d. If I couldn't locate the owner, I'd put it in the family piggy bank so I could get my loved ones something they've been saving for.

   e. Smirk at the money, thinking, "Who has money just falling out of their pocket?"

7. **Why do you think you struggle with weight loss?**

   a. I overindulge on food, then severely restrict myself. So I'm ei-ther on a diet or off the wagon, and I find myself going back and forth between them too much.

   b. I'm not sure, but I know my eating may be out of control because I never pay attention to portions or even what's in the foods I'm eating.

   c. I enjoy the social aspect of eating and sharing food with friends, though sometimes I get caught up in the experience and lose track of how much I eat.

   d. I eat carelessly when I'm around food and don't have any guide-lines to follow. But if I'm not around food, I don't really think about it so I end up missing meals.

   e. When I don't lose weight, I give up completely for a long period of time.

8. **If you overheard your close friends talking about you, what do you think they'd be saying?**

   a. I'm a bit of a leader, because I take charge, think fast, talk fast, and plan activities for the rest of our circle of friends.

   b. Endearing, lovable, and steadfast as a friend but often frustrat-ing because I'm always on my own timetable.

   c. My energy is unpredictable because it goes along with my mood, but my friends like to do things with me because I'm always up for adventure!

d. I'm exceptional at staying connected, but I could use some of the time I spend on them to spend on myself. Ultimately, they worry about my well-being in that way, and I know they're probably right!

e. I'm a bit guarded in that I have it in me to achieve my goals, if only I could get myself into gear.

9. **Getting it done? This is my style:**

a. I'll start a project and not even look at the clock till I'm done. If it's cupcakes for a bake sale or a questionnaire, I latch on and don't let go.

b. I'm great at starting, but it's finishing that drives me nuts. I have a résumé full of half-started amazing plans.

c. Unless I'm working with someone, there is no way this is going to happen. I need someone both to help and keep me accountable.

d. I do things in fits and starts. I need to snack, stretch, text, or take bathroom breaks, so it takes a while to finish, but I do.

e. Why is it so tough for me to get started on something? I *know* I'm capable of more, but I just keep talking myself out of taking the first step.

10. **You get invited to a buffet. What's your reaction?**

a. I'll go with a game plan in order to make well-balanced selections.

b. I usually eat whatever I want, so I'll just have a mishmash of what's there.

c. Why not?! Can't remember the last time I was at one of these!

d. I can't remember the last time I ate today—so a buffet sounds good and I will just try to control portions.

e. Excited to eat without limits, but I'm already anticipating the guilt I'll feel afterward.

11. **When you have a "cheat" meal, what does it look like?**

   a. My cheats are any deviation from healthy eating, no matter how small. An extra serving, even a Hershey's kiss, is a cheat to me.

   b. It's not cheating. I'm just celebrating life in the moment!

   c. Cheating is a reward after working hard in a spin class or other workout, or an excuse to go off my diet because of someone's birthday or other celebration.

   d. True cheats are big indulgences, just diving into a quart of ice cream or a package of cookies. Little cheats? They're no big deal. I need little treats sometimes to get through the day.

   e. A cheat? It's more just my way of life. But I do have my moments when I'm eating more clean.

12. **When it comes to making New Year's resolutions, yours sound like this:**

   a. I'm going to start the year on a new schedule that has a plan with clearly defined goals.

   b. I'm all about working on myself! . . . I just struggle with what to focus on.

   c. In January, my resolution might be to go to a new fitness class twice a week for a year, but by month's end, I'll be ready to switch to a different class.

   d. I'd like to start a diet and exercise program but have this gnawing feeling hanging over me that I have to somehow work my resolutions around family and other commitments.

   e. I don't make resolutions. I'll probably just peter out like I did the last time I made them.

13. **When it comes to toilet paper, what do you like best?**

   a. I like to be cost effective and stick to the same brands.

   b. I just grab Kleenex or toilet paper—whatever is there or the most convenient.

c. I go back and forth—toilet paper, Kleenex, wet wipes; they're all fine with me.

d. I prefer the softest toilet paper possible. It's a little thing that I love, plus I want my family and visitors to feel taken care of.

e. I don't give it much thought. It goes down the toilet anyway.

14. **When you're invited to something new, how "game" are you?**

a. I need to know if it's going to fit into my day or my plans first.

b. I'm game for anything; let's go now!

c. Who else is going? I'm up for anything. I'll go if you go.

d. I can go as long as I get the chores done. But are they ever done?

e. It really depends on what it is. I'm open to a lot of things, but if I don't like it I'd rather be doing something else.

15. **What kind of clothes shopper are you?**

a. I always tend to buy five of the same shirt/outfit, but in different colors. I stick to the same two or three stores.

b. I have enough clothes to fill two wardrobes and three chests of drawers . . . but I'm always on the lookout for something fun to wear.

c. I'll buy anything that's brand-new or trendy. I love discovering new and different stores.

d. I rarely go shopping unless I need something for an event or a trip. By the time I buy something, I have decided that it is something I really want. I would never buy anything just for the sake of it.

e. I do a lot of shopping but it's mostly online. I really dislike shopping in person, so if my clothes get too tight, I just order a larger size.

16. **When you clean your house or office, what's your strategy?**

   a. I like to go room by room. Systematic completion fuels my cleaning frenzy.

   b. Unless my path is disrupted, I let it pile up and just wait for a tipping point. If I can't find the other shoe in a pair or I run out of clean silverware, I know it's time to straighten up that area of the house.

   c. I start with good intentions, but I get distracted with other things I'd rather do and put it off, so I ultimately never finish.

   d. I'm focused on everything in efficient groupings to stretch my time as far as I can—I will wipe down all the countertops, then vacuum all the carpets, then clean all the mirrors, and so on.

   e. I'll take a stab at some housework; it seems like it never gets done, though, so I'll complete it halfheartedly.

17. **What happens when you're heading out and run out of clean underwear?**

   a. Really? Who runs out of underwear?

   b. I go commando—less to worry about.

   c. I head straight to my favorite underwear store and buy a pack in different colors. I love any chance I get to shop.

   d. I put on a bathing suit bottom; it will get me through the day.

   e. Ugh . . . I'll figure something out, but why does everything have to be such a project?

18. **Your boss calls in sick and tells you to take the day off, too—what would you do?**

   a. Run a bunch of errands around town and then work on something around my home that I've been dying to organize, like the pantry or a couple of closets.

   b. Thank goodness—a day to get caught up!!

   c. I'd throw myself into a fun little day—the movies, shopping, and/or dining out!

d. I would fill my day with much-needed quality time visiting with friends and family or even a phone call to a longtime bestie to get caught up.

e. Just dial back at home and relax—finally a day with nothing to do and no one to answer to.

19. **When you're feeling stressed, how does it manifest?**

a. Unconscious tics. Whether you're biting your nails, peeling off nail polish, or fidgeting, you catch yourself doing these things without even knowing you began doing them.

b. Major fatigue. You need to crash and/or shut it down for a short while.

c. Denial. You don't want to believe it, so it simply becomes untrue or you mitigate the reality in your mind.

d. Sublimate/displace energy elsewhere. You opt to stay busy, or even go harder.

e. Emotional and sometimes volatile lash-outs. They can surface in an argument or even through road rage. It comes out almost uncontrollably, "from out of nowhere," but it really stems from your unaddressed seeds of stress.

20. **You're getting your palm read and she's spot on when she describes you as:**

a. Organized and logical; you need process and order.

b. Spontaneous and fun-loving; you are always a bit disjointed.

c. Sociable and diverse; you struggle to achieve consistency.

d. Supportive but often to a fault; you love being a caregiver.

e. Effective when you choose to be but fear distorts your process; you are very communicative.

Now, go back through your answers, counting up your number of answers per letter, to identify your diet personality type. Keep in mind that there will be some outliers because as a unique human being with a complex personality, you will find yourself connected to personality characteristics that are outside your dominant findings.

Mostly A:	You are an ORGANIZED DOER.
Mostly B:	You are a REBEL.
Mostly C:	You are a SWINGER.
Mostly D:	You are an EVERYDAY HERO.
Mostly E:	You are a NEVER-EVER.

Now, when you add up your answers, you may find that next in line from your dominant answer and therefore your dominant diet personality is another personality type that had 6 or more of that letter circled; if so, you have a recessive diet personality type as well. For example, when I took the assessment I scored 12 for Everyday Hero, 6 for Organized Doer, 1 for Rebel, and 1 for Swinger. My diet personality type is Everyday Hero; however, with a score of 6, I also have a recessive diet personality of Organized Doer! When I saw this, it made so much sense to me, and I loved how all my Virgo tendencies were picked up on. The Everyday Hero plan is optimal for me because although some components of the Organized Doer plan are important for me to read, the plan itself would not be well suited for my dominant personality.

If you also find yourself with a dominant and recessive diet personality, I'm assigning you to your dominant plan; however, be sure to study the chapter about your recessive personality, especially where I discuss the qualities that encourage weight loss and weight gain—you will find some for your behaviors in there and will benefit from the extra support. As I said early on, this is not a one-size-fits-all program, so dive in to the information and support that's there.

WHAT'S NEXT?

Now that you've pinpointed your diet personality type, you are on the verge of creating life-altering change. Your mind-set is ready, you know you need to embrace your individuality and body type, and now you'll learn how to adapt everything in a way that will just *feel* like it was meant for you. The first step is to find the chapter that corresponds to your personality type. It will include everything you need, from strategies to your exact meal plan.

I designed this book so that you could finally find a plan that fits your lifestyle and personality. As I've mentioned, what works for you won't necessarily work for your friends or family members.

But I also believe that you can help others become healthier, even if you know nothing about diet and fitness. When you read the chapters, you may notice traits that seem a little too familiar. Maybe they sound like your mom or your co-worker.

I can't tell you how often people tell me their mom or sister or spouse desperately needs to lose weight and they want to help them but don't know how. So many others share your frustration, with each person looking for the approach that feels like it was made for them. As you find the program that will change your life, feel free to share what you've learned with the people in your life closest to you.

In each of the following chapters, I list for you the primary characteristics of your individual personality type, including how you act at home and work, and I define your relationship to food, diets, and exercise: a big-picture view of your personality. Once you're familiar with your personality, specifically how it relates to diet and exercise, you will find a unique four-week diet plan designed especially for you—one that fits your personality and therefore increases your chances of lasting success in weight control.

PART 2

THE PERSONALITY PLANS

CHAPTER 5

THE ORGANIZED DOER

YOUR PERSONALITY SNAPSHOT

> Excellent at homework and follow-through
> Organized
> Results-oriented
> Methodical and decisive
> Forward thinking (usually ten steps ahead of everyone else)
> Crave routine, rules, and planning
> Limited nutritional variety—content with same old, same old meals; love consistency
> Great at reading food labels, counting calories, and measuring portions
> All in or all out when it comes to diet and exercise
> Self-critical and extremely hard on yourself
> Neglect to celebrate your success or progress

Hello, Organized Doer! There's really not much standing in the way of you and a better body. You love to create an environment that is structured (think regular meals), scheduled (how about meetings at weight-loss club every Thursday?), and slow and methodical (no quick fixes, the latest celebrity diet, or gastric bypass surgery). You're highly organized and plan ahead. You're goal- and results-oriented (which people admire), you're slightly high-strung, and you dislike waste—whether of your time or food. You're great at planning and working on your plan, including diet and exercise plans. I'm willing to bet that if you work out, you have a fitness diary that records your exercise milestones and logs your progress.

In work and in life, you prefer to know exactly what's happening and when. You plan several days in advance, develop new schedules and routines that get things done more effectively, enjoy instruction manuals, hold firm opinions, love detail, and see yourself as dependable and reliable.

Okay, with all those amazing traits, why aren't you at your ideal size and shape? Maybe you committed to achieving your goal, then tried for a while, even narrowing the gap on that goal, but ultimately gave up before making it to the finish line. And, as a result, cheated yourself out of gaining a healthy, active, fun lifestyle?

I know you've tried very hard to get in shape, but your effort is not the issue—instead it's where you're placing those efforts and whether you're placing them effectively, because you don't always understand what you're doing or not doing to find success.

Often this results in you running hard in the wrong direction, without even knowing it! But don't worry, my plan for you will direct you toward tangible results—a great motivator for you. So let's take a closer look at everything you've got going on.

You are a true type A who knows it all. You thrive on completion and are transactional in nature, enjoying organization, supervision, and leadership. You're also excellent at following instructions; this brings you peace of mind, especially when you're given the correct strategy so you can execute it properly.

All of these traits serve you well at work, where I'd recognize you immediately.

If I visited your office, for example, I'd see you hunched over your desk, concentrating on an important project. Your desk is organized, not a pencil holder or paper clip out of place. I may not see any papers or forms; they're probably all neatly filed away. In general, your workspace reflects a clean and efficient environment.

You check your e-mail at specific times of the day, so that you don't get distracted or have to deal with too many interruptions. If you let me look inside your wallet, I'd see your bills in descending numerical order and all the fronts facing the same way!

Your relationship with co-workers or clients is businesslike and task-oriented. You prefer that they give you facts and data so that you and your team can make the correct decision. Your mantra is "Let's finish the job and finish it right." When running a meeting, you stick to the agenda and don't let people chitchat their way off course.

You're excellent at following instructions from superiors; this gives them peace of mind, because you execute projects thoroughly and with a quality outcome.

Likewise, your home is neat and uncluttered. Your pantry is beautifully organized—cans (with labels turned outward) are on their own shelves, as are cereals, grains, and spices. Your fridge is the same—condiments in the side compartments, fruits and veggies in their respective bins, and so forth. You never have to root around for what you need, because there's a place for everything, and everything is in its place. I wouldn't be surprised if your closet is organized, with clothes hung securely on their hangers and perhaps even color coded.

When you make plans for social events or trips, you have the itinerary mapped out to the minute. There's little room for spontaneity. You want to make sure everything runs smoothly, without surprises—including getting your kids to their activities on time.

You're excellent at making to-do lists, too, and you always use a shopping list when headed to the supermarket. The only thing you enjoy more than working off your lists is the feeling you have when crossing completed items off them!

You have a ritual for how you start your day, and it rarely varies: have a shower, brush your teeth, drink a cup of coffee or tea, get dressed, eat breakfast, and head to work. Your evening is typically the same, too: fix dinner, watch TV, unwind, walk the dog, get ready for bed, hit the sack. You just love the stabilizing structure of routine.

Now about food: undereating is often what encourages your weight gain, along with your self-criticism that is streaming constantly, all day long. Work, relationships, food choice, appearance . . . nothing is safe from the internal ridicule.

You're also a creature of habit. You like to eat the *exact same* things at the *exact same* times every day. The problem with this is that you leave little room for nutritional variety and you may be skimping on some nutrients. You've got to incorporate more variety because your diet tends to be humdrum.

You'll do best on a diet that is highly structured, with prescribed foods and recipes to eat at each meal. As long as the menu plan is somewhat tasty and clear on preparation, you're satisfied.

Of any personality, you're most likely to trade in one extreme for another. I've seen Organized Doers go from being overweight, drinking, smoking, and eating out in excess to working out at five a.m. and training for marathons, going well over in the weekly mileage, all while severely undereating. It takes a while for you to trust others, but once you do, your trust is theirs. But you don't need any hand-holding. That's because you're driven, prompt, and independent, although it's important that you don't cross the line to isolation.

AN ORGANIZED DOER IN REAL LIFE: SARAH

Sarah had weight problems all her life. "When I was about thirteen years old, my mom took me to her exercise class," she said. "But I ate so much junk food and fast food that it didn't help." Sarah put on more weight as a teenager, and in her early twenties, she took up smoking in an attempt to control her weight. Smoking became as much a bad habit as her fast-food-heavy diet, binge eating, and total lack of exercise.

By the time Sarah was in her midforties, she was a good fifty to sixty pounds overweight. Normally in control of herself at work—she is a computer programmer—Sarah had reeled out of control with her body and health. "I hated what I saw in the mirror for too long," she said. "It became time where I needed do something about it."

Sarah knew that becoming more active was going to be key to losing weight—and true to her Organized Doer personality, she also knew that setting exercise goals would be important. Her first goal was to take light walk/jogs around her neighborhood, then she graduated to doing at least three thirty-minute cardio workouts (treadmill or stair climber) each week. Dropping fifteen pounds in a month opened her mind up to believing that more could be possible if she just kept at it. Her next goal was to run a half marathon, so she threw herself into training—almost obsessively. Thankfully, she quit smoking and did it systematically with a quit-smoking seminar at a local hospital.

Sarah did run that half marathon, and later that year she completed her first full marathon—she discovered the thrill of competing—but she struggled to even finish by walking to the finish line. Something just wasn't working—and this was what led her to me. She asked me to take her on and train her. While I know she came to me in the hope of my helping her out of her slump and providing nutritional and exercise guidance, it was as much my focus to restore overall balance to her life.

I could see Sarah as an Organized Doer right away: she wore the same pair of shoes, the same brand of socks, the same black capri leggings, and one of four sports tops she owns that are identical in style, just different in color. She was always on time. I couldn't pay that girl to be late!

As an Organized Doer, Sarah followed instructions well and was very teachable. I remember one day in which I asked her to get on the treadmill for a couple of minutes to start getting warmed up. At two minutes on the nose, she jumped off the treadmill.

"What are you doing?" I asked.

"You said 'a couple of minutes'!" I was amused and amazed by how literally she took all of my instructions. When we strength-trained, Sarah counted her own reps—I didn't need to—accurately and consistently.

Sarah remained puzzled, however, by her inability to lose the rest of her weight—she had about eighteen pounds to go. She ran forty-five to sixty minutes six to seven days a week, weight-trained four times a week, and believed her diet was healthy, yet she wasn't losing weight.

One afternoon Sarah and I met for lunch. She ordered black coffee, water with lemon, and a salad topped with chicken breasts with no dressing. She didn't even finish the chicken. I offered her a few bites of what I was eating, but she refused because it had "carbs in it."

"What do you mean?" I said, confused. "What's wrong with carbs?"

"Carbs make you fat," she said.

I explained to her the fallout of that myth—and how she needed carbs to help burn fat and fuel her training, especially if she wanted to be a successful marathoner. I added that eating carb calories doesn't make the body more likely to store fat but helps your body work more effectively, allowing it to drop fat.

Then I got blunt: "You've traded in the extremes of binge eating and never moving your body to physically breaking yourself down on a daily basis. You're restricting nourishment to try to control your weight, and it's not working."

I knew that altering her diet and eating habits would be key if she wanted to get to her goal weight and achieve more staying power in future marathons. She was simply undereating and overtraining—a bad combination that would ultimately tear down her muscles and ruin her performance and overall quality of life. The obsessive exercising is characteristic of Organized Doers because they are either all in (like Sarah) or all out.

When people attempt to lose weight or keep it off, especially Organized Doers, they often "white-knuckle" it. In other words, they're so desperate to lose the weight that they make choices out of fear that they'll gain it back. So they deprive themselves of desperately needed calories while training at the same level or higher—a bad combination.

We began talking about my body, my fitness level, and the way my body looks, and she shared that she was aspiring to achieve the same thing. I had to explain to her that it was possible *only* because I ate carbohydrates, healing me, nourishing me, and providing me with the physical and mental energy to participate in my day.

"Just imagine what you might be able to accomplish if you really gave your body what it needs, if you listened to your body," I added.

The conversation was a game changer. For the first time in years of training together, she took real steps in her journey. Sarah started incorporating healthy carbohydrates into meals and snacks: fruits; starchy vegetables such as sweet potatoes; and whole grains like brown rice, sprouted breads, and oatmeal. True to her personality, she wrote down everything she ate to make sure she was fueling herself properly. Sarah was thrilled when, by the day of her next marathon, she had lost those 18 extra pounds and reached a healthy weight of 136 pounds—and she placed in the top ten of her division, her best performance to date.

"I felt amazing!" she told me.

Understanding how food really interacts with the body was truly powerful for her and started her on the successful next chapter of her wellness journey. We would still train once or twice a month just to check in and help her stay on track by feeling accountable to me. In addition, Sarah began taking other classes on her own, including boxing and Pilates, and she continues to do so to this day. She's a dream come true for a trainer, and her lifestyle-changing success is the ultimate goal I have for everyone—including you.

THE SUPPORT YOU NEED TO SUCCEED

You do well when actions and solutions are streamlined, especially because you have a "just tell me what I need to do and I'll do it" attitude. You'll be given clear expectations to follow, but I also want you celebrating your victories, no matter how big or small, along the way. For example, when you hit your highest treadmill speed in a boot camp class, don't overlook the victory and only focus on how many people ran faster than you. Don't achieve your fastest mile time ever and not celebrate it just because other people ran the entire mile whereas you needed to walk during parts of yours. Celebrate the fact that you went to dinner and didn't order dessert, for goodness' sake! You tend to brush off these achievements. Don't do it, for they will become the fuel to your weight-loss longevity. Moral of the story? When you experience success, you must celebrate it!

Setting healthy boundaries will keep you from bouncing from one extreme to another. Balance is everything! Every day, I will provide you with a little nutritional variety. However, routine is the foundation of success for you, so I will give you one. I will intentionally use similar ingredients on back-to-back nights so that grocery shopping will also be clear-cut as well.

BEHAVIOR THAT ENCOURAGES WEIGHT GAIN

- An "I'll figure it out as I go" mind-set
- Lacking direction when it comes to dieting
- Undernourishment
- Tendency to trade in old bad habits for new ones (for example, you've quit smoking but now you're a chocoholic)
- Obsessing over the scale
- Criticizing every meal and every workout
- Living in extremes

BEHAVIOR THAT ENCOURAGES WEIGHT LOSS

- Completing a daily checklist
- Tracking your water intake
- Developing a weekly schedule that can be replicated
- Executing a standard Sunday grocery list
- Nighttime rituals
- Knowing your *healthy* limits
- Zeroing in on effective training
- Competitiveness in group class settings
- Ability to celebrate successes

THE ORGANIZED DOER MEAL PLAN

Now for your plan. For starters, turn off that beautiful brain of yours and leave the thinking to me. Here, I've streamlined what you need to know and what you need to do, so you can execute the plan and thrive over the next four weeks.

You'll learn how to soften your extreme approach to nutrition and exercise, while building the confidence to live without obsessing over every bite or rep. No more living on the wagon to feel self-worth and then living off it and assigning shame. You're not built to dwell in physical or emotional highs and lows. It's just too depleting, and you end up working against your own success. This ends now.

Sharpening your self-control is the key to your success. You'll practice it over and over again on this plan through prep days, consistency in portions, and the commitment to see each daily checklist through. Just as you work your muscles in the gym, you're also going to work on your self-control so that it becomes second nature and a reliable asset.

Be aware that Day 1 for you will be just as demanding as Day 28 when it comes to my expectations on your follow-through. I did this on purpose because I know you can handle it, and I'm not willing to waste any more of your days without action. YOU ARE READY. We'll achieve a pace of weight loss and a joyful rhythm in your life that will bring not only a smile to your face but a great deal of peace to you as well.

The time is now. The focus is you. I'll meet you at the starting line.

JEN'S POWER 5 FOR ORGANIZED DOERS

1. Eat exactly what is listed—no substitutions. As an Organized Doer, you like to eat the same meals. I've structured your plan to honor that preference, but I've built in more nutritional variety for lunches and dinners.

2. Check off/highlight meals in your day as you complete them. You like to employ organizational skills in all areas of your life, and nutrition tracking is no exception, plus each notation will feel like a mini victory!

3. Batch-cook food on Sunday for Monday, Tuesday, and Wednesday; batch-cook Wednesday for Thursday, Friday, and Saturday.

4. Invest in a fun lunch sack equipped with climate control and a set of quality Tupperware that you love.

5. Follow the water-drinking schedule outlined here. Staying hydrated will keep everything moving through your system. You may perk up your water with a little lemon juice or sliced cucumbers. Also, feel free to have coffee or tea with your meals.

Sunday Preparation for Week 1

1. Wash and prep fruit and vegetables.
2. Cook chicken for wraps/freeze chicken for slow cooker.
3. Make *Tuna Salad (page 240)* (just Wednesday's portion).

Week 1 Grocery List

(Many of these ingredients you will use again in future weeks.)

PROTEIN

6 large eggs

4 boneless skinless chicken breasts

10 to 12 ounces 93% lean turkey meat

1 pork chop

2 (6-ounce) whitefish fillets

2 (3-ounce) cans tuna (water packed)

PRODUCE

1 apple

1 avocado

3 cups berries (blueberries, raspberries, and blackberries)

3 cups strawberries

1 lemon

1 lime

3 pears

1 package bean sprouts

2 green bell peppers

1 package Brussels sprouts

1 package shredded cabbage

1 package shredded carrots

1 package cauliflower florets

1 bunch celery

Cucumbers (2 regular or 6 to 8 Persian)

1 head romaine lettuce

1 onion

5 ounces fresh spinach

2 medium sweet potatoes

2 tomatoes

DAIRY

1/2 gallon 2% milk

1 package sliced Cheddar or mozzarella cheese

STARCHES

1 package brown rice

1 package gluten-free brown rice/pasta

1 package tortillas (Jen's specs: pick a wrap with whole-wheat flour listed as the first ingredient)

NUTS/OILS

1 package raw almonds

1 bottle extra-virgin olive oil

1 bottle white wine vinegar

SPICES/CONDIMENTS

Salt

Pepper

Chili powder

Garlic powder

Onion powder

Cumin

Oregano

1 bottle mustard

OTHER

1 container unsweetened vanilla almond milk

1 container hummus

1 (13-ounce) jar marinara sauce

1 jar salsa

1 container (2 pounds) protein powder (Jen's specs: 1 scoop equals 18 to 23 grams protein, 7 to 10 grams carbohydrates, and less than 5 grams sugar), flavor up to you

1 can cooking spray (vegetable, coconut, or olive oil)

MONDAY

Upon waking: 12 ounces (1½ cups) water

BREAKFAST

3-Ingredient Smoothie #1 (page 213)

MIDMORNING SNACK

1 pear and 12 ounces (1½ cups) water

LUNCH

Chicken Wrap #1 (page 225)

MIDAFTERNOON SNACK
   Handful of almonds and 12 ounces (1½ cups) water

DINNER
   Baked Whitefish with Oven-Roasted Veggies (page 244)

BEFORE BEDTIME (45 MINUTES BEFORE GOING TO BED)
   12 ounces (1½ cups) water

TUESDAY

Upon waking: 12 ounces (1½ cups) water

BREAKFAST
   3-Ingredient Smoothie #2 (page 214)

MIDMORNING SNACK
   1 cup fresh berries and 12 ounces (1½ cups) water

LUNCH
   Chicken Wrap #2 (page 226)

MIDAFTERNOON SNACK
   Handful of almonds and 12 ounces (1½ cups) water

DINNER
   Butter Lettuce Fish Tacos with Spicy Apple Slaw (page 252)

BEFORE BEDTIME (45 MINUTES BEFORE GOING TO BED)
   12 ounces (1½ cups) water

WEDNESDAY

Upon waking: 12 ounces (1½ cups) water

BREAKFAST
   3-Ingredient Smoothie #1 (page 213)

MIDMORNING SNACK
   1 pear and 12 ounces (1½ cups) water

LUNCH
   Tuna Salad Wraps (page 240)

MIDAFTERNOON SNACK
Handful of almonds and 12 ounces (1½ cups) water

DINNER
Slow Cooker Chicken Fajitas (page 279) (1 serving)
1 cup cooked brown rice

BEFORE BEDTIME (45 MINUTES BEFORE GOING TO BED)
12 ounces (1½ cups) water

THURSDAY

Upon waking: 12 ounces (1½ cups) water

BREAKFAST
3-Ingredient Smoothie #2 (page 214)

MIDMORNING SNACK
1 cup fresh berries and 12 ounces (1½ cups) water

LUNCH
Chicken Wrap #3 (page 226)

MIDAFTERNOON SNACK
Handful of almonds and 12 ounces (1½ cups) water

DINNER
Turkey Meat Sauce Pasta (page 291)

BEFORE BEDTIME (45 MINUTES BEFORE GOING TO BED)
12 ounces (1½ cups) water

FRIDAY

Upon waking: 12 ounces (1½ cups) water

BREAKFAST
3-Ingredient Smoothie #1 (page 213)

MIDMORNING SNACK
1 pear and 12 ounces (1½ cups) water

LUNCH
Tuna Salad Wraps (page 240)

MIDAFTERNOON SNACK
Handful of almonds and 12 ounces (1½ cups) water

DINNER
*Lettuce-Wrapped Turkey Burger with Baked Sweet Potato
(page 264)*

BEFORE BEDTIME (45 MINUTES BEFORE GOING TO BED)
12 ounces (1½ cups) water

SATURDAY

Upon waking: 12 ounces (1½ cups) water

BREAKFAST
3-Ingredient Smoothie #2 (page 214)

MIDMORNING SNACK
1 cup fresh berries and 12 ounces (1½ cups) water

LUNCH
Egg Salad (page 228) (on arugula)

MIDAFTERNOON SNACK
Handful of almonds and 12 ounces (1½ cups) water

DINNER
Grilled Pork and Peppers with Creamy Sweet Potato Mash (page 262)

BEFORE BEDTIME (45 MINUTES BEFORE GOING TO BED)
12 ounces (1½ cups) water

SUNDAY

Upon waking: 12 ounces (1½ cups) water

BREAKFAST
3-Ingredient Smoothie #1 (page 213)

MIDMORNING SNACK
1 apple and 12 ounces (1½ cups) water

LUNCH/BRUNCH
Cheese and Spinach Omelet (page 198)

MIDAFTERNOON SNACK
Handful of almonds and 12 ounces (1½ cups) water

DINNER
Pan-Seared Skirt Steak and Veg (page 273)

BEFORE BEDTIME (45 MINUTES BEFORE GOING TO BED)
12 ounces (1½ cups) water

WEEK 2

Sunday Preparation for Week 2
1. Make *Protein Pancakes (page 210)*.
2. Boil eggs for the week.
3. Wash and prep fruit and vegetables.
4. Make *Salmon Burgers on Butter Lettuce (page 236)* (just the patties) for lunches.
5. Cook chicken for lunches.

Week 2 Grocery List
(Many of these ingredients may be left over from Week 1. Recheck your stash before buying more.)

Note: Purchase Week 1 Sunday dinner ingredients *today* for tonight!

PROTEIN
6 large eggs

1 small container liquid egg whites

2 boneless skinless chicken breasts

12 ounces 93% lean turkey meat

6 ounces 90% lean ground beef (pick out your burger fixings, too)

6 ounces skirt steak

1 (6-ounce) halibut fillet

3 (5-ounce) salmon fillets

6 ounces precooked shrimp

1 (5-ounce) can tuna (water packed)

PRODUCE

2 Granny Smith apples

1 banana

2 cups strawberries

2 lemons

1 bundle asparagus

1 bundle broccolini

1 garlic head

5 ounces fresh kale

1 package butter lettuce (for wraps)

1 package mixed greens

1 bundle green onions (scallions)

5 ounces fresh spinach

1 medium sweet potato

2 tomatoes

DAIRY

1 tub cottage cheese

1 package feta cheese crumbles

STARCHES

1 package almond flour

1 package buckwheat flour

NUTS/OILS

1 package cashews

1 package pine nuts

1 package walnuts

1 bottle balsamic vinaigrette

SPICES/CONDIMENTS

None

OTHER

1 jar pesto

1 can cooking spray (vegetable, coconut, or olive oil)

Note: Pick two green veggies and a protein for your Friday stir-fry!

MONDAY

Upon waking: 12 ounces (1¹/₂ cups) water

BREAKFAST
2 *Protein Pancakes (page 210)*

MIDMORNING SNACK
2 hard-boiled eggs, lightly salted, and 16 ounces (2 cups) water

LUNCH
Chicken Spinach Salad (page 225)

MIDAFTERNOON SNACK
Handful of nuts (cashews or walnuts) and 16 ounces (2 cups) water

DINNER
Baked Garlic-Lemon Salmon with Herbed Brown Rice and Asparagus (page 242)

BEFORE BEDTIME (45 MINUTES BEFORE GOING TO BED)
16 ounces (2 cups) water

TUESDAY

Upon waking: 12 ounces (1 1/2 cups) water

BREAKFAST
Green Smoothie (page 219)

MIDMORNING SNACK
1/2 to 2/3 cup cottage cheese and 16 ounces (2 cups) water

LUNCH
Salmon Burgers on Butter Lettuce (page 236)

MIDAFTERNOON SNACK
Handful of nuts (cashews or walnuts) and 16 ounces (2 cups) water

DINNER
The Kale Salad (page 232) (protein addition optional)

BEFORE BEDTIME (45 MINUTES BEFORE GOING TO BED)
16 ounces (2 cups) water

WEDNESDAY

Upon waking: 12 ounces (1¹/₂ cups) water

BREAKFAST
  2 *Protein Pancakes (page 210)*

MIDMORNING SNACK
  2 hard-boiled eggs, lightly salted, and 16 ounces (2 cups) water

LUNCH
  Chicken Spinach Salad (page 225)

MIDAFTERNOON SNACK
  Handful of nuts (cashews or walnuts) and 16 ounces (2 cups)
    water

DINNER
  Turkey Burger Sammie with Chopped Kale Salad (page 290)

BEFORE BEDTIME (45 MINUTES BEFORE GOING TO BED)
  16 ounces (2 cups) water

THURSDAY

Upon waking: 12 ounces (1¹/₂ cups) water

BREAKFAST
  Green Smoothie (page 219)

MIDMORNING SNACK
  ¹/₂ to ²/₃ cup cottage cheese and 16 ounces (2 cups) water

LUNCH
  Chicken Spinach Salad (page 225)

MIDAFTERNOON SNACK
  Handful of nuts (cashews or walnuts) and 16 ounces (2 cups)
    water

DINNER
  Shrimp Pasta (page 277)

BEFORE BEDTIME (45 MINUTES BEFORE GOING TO BED)
16 ounces (2 cups) water

FRIDAY

Upon waking: 12 ounces (1¹/₂ cups) water

BREAKFAST
2 *Protein Pancakes (page 210)*

MIDMORNING SNACK
2 hard-boiled eggs, lightly salted, and 16 ounces (2 cups) water

LUNCH
Salmon Burgers on Butter Lettuce (page 236)

MIDAFTERNOON SNACK
Handful of nuts (cashews or walnuts) and 16 ounces (2 cups) water

DINNER
DIY Stir-Fry (page 254) (make two portions so you're set for lunch tomorrow)

BEFORE BEDTIME (45 MINUTES BEFORE GOING TO BED)
16 ounces (2 cups) water

SATURDAY

Upon waking: 12 ounces (1¹/₂ cups) water

BREAKFAST
2 *Protein Pancakes (page 210)*

MIDMORNING SNACK
2 hard-boiled eggs, lightly salted, and 16 ounces (2 cups) water

LUNCH
DIY Stir-Fry (page 254) (left over from Friday)

MIDAFTERNOON SNACK
Handful of nuts (cashews or walnuts) and 16 ounces (2 cups) water

DINNER
Zucchini Pesto Pasta Sauté (page 293) (with 6 ounces ground turkey)

BEFORE BEDTIME (45 MINUTES BEFORE GOING TO BED)
16 ounces (2 cups) water

SUNDAY

Upon waking: 12 ounces (1½ cups) water

BREAKFAST
Green Smoothie (page 219)

MIDMORNING SNACK
½ to ⅔ cup cottage cheese and 16 ounces (2 cups) water

LUNCH/BRUNCH
Tuna Salad (page 240) (on spinach)

MIDAFTERNOON SNACK
Handful of nuts (cashews or walnuts) and 16 ounces (2 cups) water

DINNER
Burger Bowl (page 250)

BEFORE BEDTIME (45 MINUTES BEFORE GOING TO BED)
16 ounces (2 cups) water

WEEK 3

Sunday Preparation for Week 3

1. Make *Egg Salad (page 228)*.

2. Prep butter lettuce for lunches.

3. Wash and prep fruit and vegetables.

Week 3 Grocery List

(Many of these ingredients may be left over from Weeks 1 and 2. Recheck your stash before buying more.)

PROTEIN

12 large eggs

4 boneless skinless chicken breasts

6 ounces skirt steak

6 ounces whitefish

6 ounces cooked shrimp

1 (5-ounce) can tuna (water packed)

PRODUCE

5 apples

4 avocados

2 bananas

1 small container of berries (blueberries, raspberries, or blackberries)

1 small container of strawberries

3 lemons

2 orange or yellow bell peppers

1 bunch celery

2 ears of corn

1 cucumber

1 garlic clove

1 head butter lettuce

1 head romaine lettuce

1 package fresh spinach

1 medium sweet potato

2 pints cherry tomatoes

12 ounces green beans

DAIRY

1/2 gallon 2% milk or unsweetened vanilla almond milk

1 package shredded mozzarella cheese

1 small block Parmesan cheese

STARCHES

1 container old-fashioned oats (Jen's specs: contains 5 grams or more of fiber and under 10 grams of sugar per cooked serving)

1 box granola (Jen's specs: contains 5 grams or more of fiber and under 10 grams of sugar per serving)

NUTS/OILS
1 small package macadamia
nuts

SPICES/CONDIMENTS
None

OTHER
1 small package chia seeds   1 roll of aluminum foil

MONDAY

Upon waking: 12 ounces (1½ cups) water

BREAKFAST
Oatmeal Granola Combo (page 207)

MIDMORNING SNACK
1 apple and 20 ounces (2½ cups) water

LUNCH
Egg Salad (page 228) wraps (I suggest using butter lettuce or
romaine leaves)

MIDAFTERNOON SNACK
½ avocado with lemon and salt and 20 ounces (2½ cups) water

DINNER
Grilled Herbed Chicken with Spicy String Beans (page 260)

BEFORE BEDTIME (60 MINUTES BEFORE GOING TO BED)
20 ounces (2½ cups) water

TUESDAY

Upon waking: 12 ounces (1½ cups) water

BREAKFAST
5-Ingredient Smoothie (page 214)

MIDMORNING SNACK
1 banana and 20 ounces (2¹/₂ cups) water

LUNCH
Chopped Romaine Salad with Herbed Vinaigrette (page 227)

MIDAFTERNOON SNACK
¹/₂ avocado with lemon and salt and 20 ounces (2¹/₂ cups) water

DINNER
Foil-Wrapped Fish 1.0 (page 257)
Leftover green beans from Monday

BEFORE BEDTIME (60 MINUTES BEFORE GOING TO BED)
20 ounces (2¹/₂ cups) water

WEDNESDAY

Upon waking: 12 ounces (1¹/₂ cups) water

BREAKFAST
Oatmeal Granola Combo (page 207)

MIDMORNING SNACK
1 apple and 20 ounces (2¹/₂ cups) water

LUNCH
Egg Salad (page 228) wraps (I suggest using butter lettuce or
romaine leaves)

MIDAFTERNOON SNACK
¹/₂ avocado with lemon and salt and 20 ounces (2¹/₂ cups) water

DINNER
*Slow Cooker Turkey Meatballs with Baked Sweet Potato "Chips"
(page 282)*

BEFORE BEDTIME (60 MINUTES BEFORE GOING TO BED)
20 ounces (2¹/₂ cups) water

THURSDAY

Upon waking: 12 ounces (1½ cups) water

BREAKFAST
5-Ingredient Smoothie (page 214)

MIDMORNING SNACK
1 banana and 20 ounces (2½ cups) water

LUNCH
Chopped Romaine Salad with Herbed Vinaigrette (page 227) plus
5 leftover turkey meatballs

MIDAFTERNOON SNACK
½ avocado with lemon and salt and 20 ounces (2½ cups) water

DINNER
DIY Stir-Fry (page 254) (with 6 ounces shrimp)

BEFORE BEDTIME (60 MINUTES BEFORE GOING TO BED)
16 ounces (2½ cups) water

FRIDAY

Upon waking: 12 ounces (1½ cups) water

BREAKFAST
Oatmeal Granola Combo (page 207)

MIDMORNING SNACK
1 apple and 20 ounces (2½ cups) water

LUNCH
Egg Salad (page 228) wraps (I suggest using butter lettuce or
romaine leaves)

MIDAFTERNOON SNACK
½ avocado with lemon and salt and 20 ounces (2½ cups) water

DINNER
Mama Widerstrom's Grilled Caesar Salad with Skirt Steak (page 266)

BEFORE BEDTIME (60 MINUTES BEFORE GOING TO BED)
20 ounces (2$\frac{1}{2}$ cups) water

SATURDAY

Upon waking: 12 ounces (1$\frac{1}{2}$ cups) water

BREAKFAST
5-Ingredient Smoothie (page 214)

MIDMORNING SNACK
1 banana and 20 ounces (2$\frac{1}{2}$ cups) water

LUNCH
Tuna Salad (page 240) (on spinach and/or romaine lettuce)

MIDAFTERNOON SNACK
$\frac{1}{2}$ avocado with lemon and salt and 20 ounces (2$\frac{1}{2}$ cups) water

DINNER
Eggplant Parmesan (page 255)

BEFORE BEDTIME (60 MINUTES BEFORE GOING TO BED)
16 ounces (2$\frac{1}{2}$ cups) water

SUNDAY

Upon waking: 12 ounces (1$\frac{1}{2}$ cups) water

BREAKFAST
Oatmeal Granola Combo (page 207)

MIDMORNING SNACK
1 apple and 20 ounces (2$\frac{1}{2}$ cups) water

LUNCH/BRUNCH
Scrambled Egg Veggie Breakfast Burrito (page 210)

MIDAFTERNOON SNACK
$\frac{1}{2}$ avocado with lemon and salt and 20 ounces (2$\frac{1}{2}$ cups) water

DINNER
One-Pot Chicken (page 269)

BEFORE BEDTIME (60 MINUTES BEFORE GOING TO BED)
16 ounces (2 cups) water

WEEK 4

Sunday Preparation for Week 4

1. Prepare *Banana Walnut Muffins (page 197)*.
2. Wash and prep fruit and vegetables.
3. Freeze blueberries.
4. Cook chicken for wraps.
5. Cook quinoa.

Week 4 Grocery List

(Many of these ingredients may be left over from Weeks 1, 2, and 3. Recheck your stash before buying more.)

PROTEIN

12 large eggs

5 boneless skinless chicken breasts

6 ounces 93% lean ground turkey

6 ounces 90% lean ground beef

6 ounces steak filet

6 ounces salmon fillet

PRODUCE

1 apple

2 avocados

1 banana

1 pint blueberries

2 lemons

4 cups pineapple chunks

1 bundle asparagus

1 package basil

1 green bell pepper

2 packages precut broccoli florets

1 package shredded cabbage

1 (16-ounce) package baby carrots

6 to 8 Persian cucumbers

2 packages fresh kale

1 head romaine lettuce

1 bundle green onions (scallions)

5 ounces fresh spinach

1 medium sweet potato

1 pint cherry tomatoes

1 zucchini

DAIRY

4 cups 2% Greek yogurt

1 package natural, hard
cheese (Cheddar,
mozzarella, Swiss, or
Parmesan)

STARCHES

1 package quinoa

NUTS/OILS

1 package sliced almonds

SPICES/CONDIMENTS

1 bottle low-sodium soy
sauce

OTHER

1 package golden raisins

1 package hummus

1 package tzatziki sauce

1 bottle chipotle pepper
sauce

1 bottle maple syrup

1 can cooking spray
(vegetable, coconut, or
olive oil)

Muffin pan

MONDAY

Upon waking: 16 ounces (2 cups) water

BREAKFAST
Green Omelet (page 204)

MIDMORNING SNACK
1 cup pineapple chunks and 24 ounces (3 cups) water

LUNCH
The Kale Salad (page 232) (omit protein)

MIDAFTERNOON SNACK
4 to 6 tablespoons hummus with carrots and cucumbers for
dipping and 24 ounces (3 cups) water

DINNER
Oven-Baked Salmon with Roasted Brussels Sprouts and Almonds
(page 271)

BEFORE BEDTIME (60 MINUTES BEFORE GOING TO BED)
20 ounces (2½ cups) water

TUESDAY

Upon waking: 16 ounces (2 cups) water

BREAKFAST
½ cantaloupe filled with 1 cup 2% Greek yogurt

MIDMORNING SNACK
2 *Banana Walnut Muffins (page 197)* and 20 ounces (2½ cups)
water

LUNCH
Chicken Wrap #2 (page 226)

MIDAFTERNOON SNACK
4 to 6 tablespoons tzatziki sauce with carrots and cucumbers for
dipping and 24 ounces (3 cups) water

DINNER
Zucchini Pesto Pasta Sauté (page 293) (with 6 ounces shrimp)

BEFORE BEDTIME (60 MINUTES BEFORE GOING TO BED)
20 ounces (2½ cups) water

WEDNESDAY

Upon waking: 16 ounces (2 cups) water

BREAKFAST
Green Omelet (page 204)

MIDMORNING SNACK
1 cup pineapple chunks and 24 ounces (3 cups) water

LUNCH
The Kale Salad (page 232) (omit protein)

MIDAFTERNOON SNACK
4 to 6 tablespoons hummus with carrots and cucumbers for
dipping and 24 ounces (3 cups) water

DINNER
*Turkey Burger with Caramelized Onion and Baked Sweet Potato
"Chips" (page 288)*

BEFORE BEDTIME (60 MINUTES BEFORE GOING TO BED)
20 ounces (2½ cups) water

THURSDAY

Upon waking: 16 ounces (2 cups) water

BREAKFAST
½ cantaloupe filled with 1 cup 2% Greek yogurt

MIDMORNING SNACK
2 *Banana Walnut Muffins (page 197)* and 20 ounces (2½ cups)
water

LUNCH
Chicken Wrap #2 (page 226)

MIDAFTERNOON SNACK
4 to 6 tablespoons tzatziki sauce with carrots and cucumbers for
dipping and 24 ounces (3 cups) water

DINNER
Soy-Honey Chicken with Broccoli (page 284)

BEFORE BEDTIME (60 MINUTES BEFORE GOING TO BED)
20 ounces (2½ cups) water

FRIDAY

Upon waking: 16 ounces (2 cups) water

BREAKFAST
Green Omelet (page 204)

MIDMORNING SNACK
1 cup pineapple chunks and 24 ounces (3 cups) water

LUNCH
The Kale Salad (page 232) (omit protein)

MIDAFTERNOON SNACK
4 to 6 tablespoons hummus with carrots and cucumbers for
dipping and 24 ounces (3 cups) water

DINNER
Butter Lettuce Fish Tacos with Spicy Apple Slaw (page 252)

BEFORE BEDTIME (60 MINUTES BEFORE GOING TO BED)
20 ounces (2$\frac{1}{2}$ cups) water

SATURDAY

Upon waking: 16 ounces (2 cups) water

BREAKFAST
Green Smoothie (page 219)

MIDMORNING SNACK
2 *Banana Walnut Muffins (page 197)* and 20 ounces (2$\frac{1}{2}$ cups)
water

LUNCH
Burger Bowl (page 250)

MIDAFTERNOON SNACK
4 to 6 tablespoons tzatziki sauce with carrots and cucumbers for
dipping and 24 ounces (3 cups) water

DINNER
  Steak and Eggs with Pan-Roasted Tomatoes (page 211)

BEFORE BEDTIME (60 MINUTES BEFORE GOING TO BED)
  20 ounces (2¹/₂ cups) water

SUNDAY

  Upon waking: 16 ounces (2 cups) water

BREAKFAST
  1 cup 2% Greek yogurt mixed with 1 cup frozen blueberries and
    ¹/₄ cup granola

MIDMORNING SNACK
  1 cup pineapple chunks and 24 ounces (3 cups) water

LUNCH/BRUNCH
  Ham and Avocado Frittata (page 205)

MIDAFTERNOON SNACK
  4 to 6 tablespoons hummus with carrots and cucumbers for
    dipping and 24 ounces (3 cups) water

DINNER
  Veggie Basil Pasta (page 292)

BEFORE BEDTIME (60 MINUTES BEFORE GOING TO BED)
  20 ounces (2¹/₂ cups) water

Meet Melanie

"My goals were simple: to be at a healthy weight but, more important, to be able to look in the mirror and not hate the sight of my own body.

"My challenges were tougher. I had been overweight for as long as I can remember. I loved food, and I have always used it for comfort. The thought of being in a gym or taking a class with normal-weight, healthy people filled me with fear and anxiety. These emotions held me back from making changes. As an Organized Doer, I hate to fail at dieting or exercising, so it was better not to try than to fail.

"I found Jen and her personality-type diet, and they changed my life. I learned about portion control and a meal plan that fit my personality (it didn't even feel like a diet!). I ate tasty food. I could go out to lunch and eat healthy, since Jen taught me how to order. The meal plan was easy to prepare, and I didn't have to buy fancy ingredients. It was tailored not only to foods I liked but also to my lifestyle.

"Jen held me accountable to this meal plan. More important, she believed I could succeed and taught me that I can't fail at this if I try my best, and that I may not always be perfect, but it's about constantly improving over time and recognizing when I fall back into old habits.

"I reached my ideal weight and have maintained it all these years later. I continue to use the personality-based tools Jen taught me in order to maintain a healthy lifestyle. I exercise regularly and eat healthy foods. Most important, I feel happy with how I look and am no longer ashamed of my body."

PEP TALK

Of all the personality types, you will see the fastest progress in your diet. This is not me exaggerating but simply stating the truth about how valuable your personality qualities are. Your love of organization will help you find a healthy rhythm and master follow-through. Execute each day with a little celebration because your success depends on it. But also call upon your work ethic as well as the connection you're developing with your body.

Do not punish yourself for any slip-ups that may occur either; simply analyze and assess any contributing variables and make the adjustment going forward. Easy peasy! By the end of these four weeks, my Organized Doer, I want you to see the grounded, capable, and special person that I see in you. Believe in that truth—starting now.

CHAPTER 6

THE SWINGER

YOUR PERSONALITY SNAPSHOT

> Open to new experiences and adventures

> Very passionate about projects at first but lose interest

> Social and extroverted—a fun friend

> Communicate expressively

> Require accountability

> Swing between "treating" and "punishing" with food, depending on what is going on in your life

> Always trying the latest diet—which can result in ups and downs in weight

> Skip around from one workout regimen to the next—never giving the exercise/workout a full shot

> Have a "seeing is believing" mind-set

> Very communicative with friends (via social media posts and e-mails) when you do well

f I went to a party or other event, I could spot you a mile away. You're the one having the most fun, right in the center of the action, telling stories, getting people to dance, and building instant rapport with everyone in the room. That's because you're outgoing and conversational, though with a "ten-second-Tom syndrome," as you skip around from topic to topic.

I'd call you the champion of "never a dull moment." You are a true adventurer who thrives on discovering new people, places, things, and ideas. Your friends, family, and co-workers frequently regard you as jumping around from place to place and from decision to decision. You often have more energy than anyone around you, but you tend to be restless and are forever changing your mind or your direction.

Your best motivator is positive inspiration, propelled by a "grit your teeth and do it" mind-set. Seeing others build killer bodies gets you thinking more optimistically. If they can do it, so can you. Once you take ownership of the possibilities, the sky is the limit. When your family, friends, and colleagues start noticing the weight loss, you're even more motivated to keep moving forward.

All these cool traits transfer to your job. You're outgoing, you're warm, and you usually have an expressive speaking style. You hate to dress blandly or too conservatively. You love doing business with people you like and respect. You enjoy networking and have a devoted pack of peers and pals. Your network tends to consist of people with different skills who can be called upon when needed. On the surface, you're the happiest out among clients and colleagues.

You know how to make your fellow workers feel important. When they do something for you, you always thank them and acknowledge their good work in front of all. You also stand by your colleagues during times of crisis.

You're highly creative on the job, often required to "think outside the box," and quite good at it, too. Frequently, however, you change your vision to accomplish goals. Some co-workers thus think you're inconsistent and unpredictable, but almost always, you get the job done. When change is needed in the workplace, you're the go-to person.

You may also be someone who has changed jobs and careers frequently, because of boredom or your restless need for change. None of this has slowed you down on your way to success. It's more invigorating to try new jobs every so often.

If invited to your home, I'd find a lovely, almost home-decor-magazine look in your house—with lots of windows, a creative but eclectic arrangement of furniture, and enticing interiors. But I might visit you again a few months later and find new pieces of furniture or see a completely rearranged room.

You bounce around from being very engaged to very bored. And you'd rather be anything but bored. Sometimes this creates conflict in your relationship, as when your partner wants to stay home and you want to go out. Changing your mind so frequently about what to do and where to go can cause strain, too.

You do your best parenting when full of energy and out in the field, involved in your kids' activities. You simply love to connect with people, whenever and wherever; being isolated at home for too long just isn't your thing.

That's why you enjoy dining out, preferably at different restaurants, rather than having a standard place to go. You're open to trying any food at least once, as long as it looks interesting and appetizing when it's served. You're most tempted by meals that are visually stimulating and different from the norm.

You don't have a standard repertoire of meal recipes, either. One night, you might serve basic herbed chicken breasts; another night, brandy steak flambé. In the kitchen, you're adventurous and experimental.

You dislike cooking for one because dining out is more fun and social. But if you're having a dinner party at your house with lots of friends and family, you go gung-ho. And no wonder: you're extroverted and full of fun, and you love the company of others.

When it comes to dieting, you're all over the map. You'll be the first to try the diet du jour or buy the latest diet best-seller. You start out with gritty determination. You buy and eat healthy food. You lose some weight but then get bored with the program and go off it, regaining the lost pounds. Back you go on another quest to find another new diet to start. I'd say you are the quintessential serial dieter. You also oscillate between treating and punishing yourself. For example, if you get a raise at work, you treat yourself to a sumptuous dinner. Afterward, feeling guilty, you might restrict your food for a couple of days as punishment.

You dislike meal planning to the point that you choose your meals in the moment based on what you feel like or on what others are eating around you. You'd rather eat what's available, healthy or not, and worry about the consequences later. A set meal plan takes the fun out of eating and dieting. You need plenty of options in order to satisfy your desires and not feel hemmed in by a strict plan. And counting calories, points, carbs, or fats? Forget about it. You don't want to morph into that boring person who lives on celery, doesn't drink wine, and has a near-fainting spell at the mere mention of fast food. You want to live! . . . But you want to be lean, too.

Grocery shopping tends to be hit-and-miss, and you often come out with a variety of items, some good and some not so good. In fact, you often make multiple trips to the grocery store each week because you want to add a fun ingredient to a recipe or you read a food blog describing a meal that you want to attempt—a habit that sets you up for tempting food purchases you don't need.

All in all, feeling a part of the community is just as important to you as your physical success story. Contemplative, creative, and inspired by what's trending, you find joy and therefore success in being immersed in a brand and fluent in the conversations revolving around it.

A SWINGER IN REAL LIFE: ASHLEY

Ashley is a delightful person. I call her "my little socialite." During our training sessions she likes to gab with me—I get all the in-town gossip from her—as well as with others in the gym. Every time she comes in for a session, she's wearing a new workout top and carrying a fabulous purse, and she somehow gets through our workout wearing jewelry. And I'm talking about some real bling!

As for training together, initially she was present in every session, although she never quite put into the workout what she was capable of. Ironically, during the sessions in which I tried to coach her more aggressively, she felt like she was maxing out, giving 1,000 percent and not able go even a hair harder. What I discovered was that she was operating under a perceived ceiling that stopped her short of her true capacity. That showed up in our routine, as well as the fact that she wasn't always consistent. Ashley would disappear on me from time to time, taking a vacation or extended hiatus because she needed "rest" or wanted to try something else with her workout. She'd try a spin studio one month, only to give up on it because it was too repetitive and the music "too loud." She'd then migrate to another exercise class, somewhere else, where the instructors were great but then she claimed the classes were "too packed." From there, Ashley would try a new trainer but didn't like his lack of energy . . . so she eventually found her way back to me.

Her behavior is so typical of Swingers. At the beginning, a program is exciting. They're interested and invested, but when their mood turns fickle, they want to move on to something else that feels new and fresh.

Along with Ashley's swinging from one type of workout to another, her weight was swinging up and down, too. "I was always searching for an accessible, foolproof way to slim down fast," she told me. "But nothing seemed to work for me." By age thirty-eight, she reached a number on the scale that she'd never seen before—all the back-and-forth weight loss and weight gain over the years finally caught up with her. With the scale at 180 pounds, she was scared to turn forty at that unhappy size.

We discussed how random dieting plans and inconsistent exercising were getting her nowhere. I offered her a program tailored to her love of change and need for variety, and she felt more motivated to put in the time and energy required for lasting weight loss. I told her she didn't have to ditch her favorite indulgences, like cocktails (a big part of her social life); she just had to quit making them an everyday habit. Ashley also cut back on her large, sugar-filled mocha lattes, deep-fried sushi, triple-decker sandwiches, and favorite baked goods—replacing them with more fruits, vegetables, whole grains, and lean proteins like fish.

For workouts, I constantly changed up the challenge—different exercises, different sequences of exercises, and so forth. Ashley never knew what I had in store for her in each session—and this variety kept her motivated. I had to push her, keeping her out of breath so she had no opportunity to gab because she was so focused on the movement and her breathing. We made progress because she was enthusiastic about undertaking a fitness journey that was suited to her. I listened to her, and because she felt heard, she became so connected to that bigger picture she always knew was there.

Before long Ashley was losing two to three pounds a week. After about four months, she was down forty pounds.

Ashley told me: "I didn't realize this could be so easy. You said the weight would come off, and I was too nervous to believe you, but it did. I feel so much more strength, and life has become so much easier now that I'm happy with myself."

THE SUPPORT YOU NEED TO SUCCEED

The big picture is too big for you, so small, measurable, daily goals are your jam. You live by the power of your word, so if you say you're going to do something, you do it. You've just got to build on the belief that you can do it. To *know* what you set out to do and actually achieve it is powerful for you—whether it's to drink 50 ounces of water a day for one week or pack a lunch for all five workdays that week and stick to it.

I will prove to you how successful you can be by being someone you yourself can count on. Education and accountability are *key* to your success in this group, as well as finding activities and plans that will truly hold your interest.

You are not someone who thrives independently. You *need* a point person and/or a system of checking in, in which there are consequences of falling short of daily and weekly commitments. Accountability could be in the form of a personal trainer, an online or app-based community, or a fitness studio that's heavily community-based. An authentic belonging and relationship will be huge for you.

BEHAVIOR THAT ENCOURAGES WEIGHT GAIN

- Bailing out of training systems too early
- Isolation
- Dishonesty with yourself
- Going into "screw it" mode
- Impatience with progress
- Avoiding the scale/ignoring increases in body and clothing size
- Lack of vulnerability
- Not enough real food/not cooking

- Having an accountability partner
- Signing up in advance for classes and training sessions
- Staying informed about what's relevant in the fitness world
- Not quitting (sticking to my four-week plan and paying for a month in advance!)
- SEEING IT AND SAYING IT! Placing a picture on your phone and/or your fridge that represents your end goal. A photo that you're proud of, happy in, your "shit, I looked good there" pic. A favorite selfie. A pic where you loved your body—that's where I'm taking you.
- Tracking your gym success
- Publicly sharing your goals
- Using fitness tracking/sharing apps

THE SWINGER MEAL PLAN

It's time you start giving yourself a little credit. Much of your energy and influence comes from outside yourself, but through this meal plan, I'll prove to you how strong and capable you truly are from within. The ever-changing menu items will keep you interested and engaged as your body starts trusting you again. It will demonstrate that trust by dropping inches and pounds from all over your physique.

I've developed an "options menu" for you because it's important that you have input into meal decisions. Therefore, I'm giving you the creative freedom to put each day together based on how you're feeling but within the guidelines that I've set for you. Varied consistency will be the magic fairy dust for you!

I do want to point out that snacking will not be on your menu, because in your world, it's often used as a filler for boredom, social agendas, or lack thereof. Without snacks, you'll quickly learn the difference between filling up for happiness versus filling up to satisfy hunger.

Also, I want you to record your weight and take starting measurements of your chest, high waist, low tummy, and booty. Then remeasure all these again at two weeks and four weeks. Building in this accountability and proof of progress will be a game-changing component for you and your weight loss.

The other major key to success on this plan will be committing to it once you've started it. You will see value not only in the decrease in your body measurements but also in the days completed with optimal meals, positive self-talk, and workouts that made you feel good.

You can absolutely do this, and it yields high results. No more letting the scale tell you how your day is going to be or allowing the rise and fall of your day to dictate your food choices. Together, we'll stay in the now—because moments make minutes, minutes make days, and with me in your corner we will string up great day after great day and make a fantastic you.

JEN'S POWER 5 FOR SWINGERS

1. Each week of your plan gives you four options for breakfast, lunch, and dinner. All you have to do is choose your breakfast option, lunch option, and dinner option each day, and you're on the road to success. You will be the one to build each day's meal plan, including the variety you crave.

   Make sure you plan out your grocery list according to your menu choices so you're not wandering down the wrong aisles at the grocery store!

2. As a serial dieter, you've put yourself down a lot when you've failed on a diet. Start countering this now. Practice self-talk through the week, because once you believe in yourself, you can accomplish anything. Make a conscious effort to ensure that every word, thought, and action is positive, and practice expressing these affirmations every chance you

get. Understand that the mind, like any muscle, increases in power the more you train and exercise it.

3. Prepare your hydration station. Get a good 18-to-24-ounce reusable nonplastic water bottle. As I help you elevate your water consumption, you'll end up going through a lot of single-use bottles' worth of water—1,976 water bottles in a year, to be exact—so let's be awesome to your body while still being awesome to the planet, okay?

   Weekly water tracking is as follows:

   Week 1: 2 fills plus 8 ounces (1 cup) upon waking each day
   Week 2: 3 fills
   Week 3: 4 fills
   Week 4: 5 fills

4. Use the buddy system! Connect with a friend, family member, or co-worker on completing daily challenges together that highlight your water consumption, without deviating from your plan and/or working out. Accountability to a counterpart in this process will massively raise your ability to stay invested and excited each day because you're not doing it on your own.

5. Stick to your menu meals—no snacking. For your personality specifically, snacks often turn into grazing from one meal to the next so you begin to unknowingly accumulate excess calories because you are essentially eating all day. Also, research shows that after snacking, some people are inclined to eat just as much at meals as they do when they don't snack. If you want to stay slim, snacking is not always the best way to do it, especially with your personality type. Because you love the sensation and pleasure of eating, you will wind up consuming more calories overall.

Hydration Station: 2 water bottle fills daily, after 8 ounces (1 cup) water upon waking each day

BREAKFAST MENU OPTIONS

Option A: *Banana Nut Protein Smoothie (page 216)*

Option B: Eggs any style plus toast

(*Example:* 2 hard-boiled eggs with 2 slices sprouted bread such as Ezekiel and 1½ teaspoons honey or agave)

Option C: *Egg and Potato Scramble (page 199)*

Option D: 1 cup 2% Greek yogurt with 2 cups strawberries and ½ cup granola (Jen's specs: contains 5 grams or more of fiber and under 10 grams of sugar per serving)

LUNCH MENU OPTIONS

Option A: *Sandwich Wrap (page 237)*

Option B: *Spinach and Pear Salad (page 239)*

Option C: *Green Detox Smoothie (page 219)*

Option D: *Creamy Butternut Squash Soup (page 228)*

DINNER MENU OPTIONS

Option A: *Farm to Sea Stir-Fry (page 256)*

Option B: *Burger Bowl (page 250)*

Option C: *Spring Greens Super Salad (page 286)*

Option D: *Gluten-Free Veggie Pasta (page 259)*

WEEK 2

Hydration Station: 3 water bottle fills daily

BREAKFAST MENU OPTIONS

Option A: *Strawberry Chocolate Protein Smoothie (page 224)*

Option B: ½ cantaloupe with 1 cup cottage cheese *or* 1 cup 2% Greek yogurt drizzled with a thin ribbon of honey or agave

Option C: *Pizza Omelet (page 208)*

Option D: *GGPs (Gluten-Free Green Pancakes) (page 202)*

LUNCH MENU OPTIONS

Option A: *Tuna Salad (page 240)* (on spinach)

Option B: *High-Protein Pita Pocket (page 231)*

Option C: *Southwest Veggie Chop (page 238)*

Option D: *Turmeric Lentil and Farro Soup (page 241)*

DINNER MENU OPTIONS

Option A: *DIY Stir-Fry (page 254)*

Option B: *Lemon Pepper Grilled Steak Salad (page 264)*

Option C: *Zucchini Pesto Pasta Sauté (page 293)* (with chicken)

Option D: *Slow Cooker Chicken Fajitas (page 279)* (in butter lettuce wraps)

WEEK 3

Hydration Station: 4 water bottle fills daily

BREAKFAST MENU OPTIONS

Option A: *Banana Berry Protein Smoothie (page 215)*

Option B: *Homemade Parfait (page 205)*

Option C: *Protein Oats 1.0 (page 209)*

Option D: *Black Bean Egg Scramble (page 198)*

LUNCH MENU OPTIONS

Option A: *Mediterranean Romaine Wraps (page 232)*

Option B: *Egg Salad (page 228)* (on arugula)

Option C: *Forever Young Smoothie (page 218)*

Option D: *Roasted Sweet Potato and Cauliflower Soup (page 234)*

DINNER MENU OPTIONS

Option A: *Strawberry Spinach Salad (page 287)*

Option B: *Butter Lettuce Fish Tacos with Spicy Apple Slaw (page 252)*

Option C: *Simple Steak Filet with Mushroom and Asparagus Quinoa (page 278)*

Option D: *Breakfast for Dinner (page 249)*

WEEK 4

Hydration Station: 5 water bottle fills daily

BREAKFAST MENU OPTIONS

Option A: *Blueberry Protein Smoothie (page 217)*

Option B: *Open-Faced Egg Sandwich (page 208)*

Option C: *Garden Omelet (page 201)*

Option D: *Oatmeal and Egg Bake (page 206)*

LUNCH MENU OPTIONS

Option A: *The Kale Salad (page 232)*

Option B: *Salmon Burgers on Butter Lettuce (page 236)*

Option C: *Shaved Brussels Sprouts Salad (page 238)*

Option D: *Hearty Minestrone Soup (page 230)*

DINNER MENU OPTIONS

Option A: *Mama Widerstrom's Grilled Caesar Salad with Skirt Steak (page 266)*

Option B: *Roasted Halibut with Veggie Medley (page 275)*
Option C: *Bison Beef Meatballs with Baked Sweet Potato (page 247)*
Option D: *Foil-Wrapped Fish 2.0 (page 258)*

Meet Tynan

"I really had some big changes to make: getting active again with a regular exercise routine, giving up junk food, and cutting back on alcoholic beverages when I was out socially. I also had to stop beating myself up over all the times I had failed to get in shape. Plus, I didn't want to let Jen and my wife down.

"Because my personality type is a Swinger, Jen had to help me nail down some concrete goals, such as the following:

- Exercise on a regular weekly basis and be active for thirty minutes each session.

- Achieve a healthier nutritional lifestyle by switching to healthier foods and beverages.

- Lose weight and get my body lean.

- Strive for baby steps (for example, while running, pick a landmark to run to, or pick a time on the treadmill to sprint to and then jog/walk). I found that achieving smaller goals helped me set and achieve larger goals, which gave me a better sense of accomplishment and drive.

- Make my plan sustainable over a long period in life and not just a blitzkrieg diet that would have me falling back into a poor routine in a month.

- Again: Not to let Jen or my wife and daughter down.

"I learned so much by following a plan matched to my personality. Although people often realize that to be healthy, you need to eat healthy, they don't truly understand what this means. There is often the misconception that eating healthy means eating only carrots and lettuce. Jen's program helped me see that I could eat a hearty portion for a meal and get full on flavor-filled, delicious foods.

"One thing that helped me tremendously was following exact meal times and the water schedule. This helped my body stay satisfied all day and kept me from eating larger meals for lunch and dinner. Having the Swinger's guideline of foods to eat helped me control portions and not swing back to unhealthy eating. I had plenty of meal options, and they were very helpful.

"The results of the Swinger meal plan: I lost nineteen pounds and four inches off my waist in my first four weeks with Jen's program! I can only imagine the drops I will experience as I continue this forward.

"Jen's personality-type diet plan has not only altered my physical appearance, but has also changed my formerly clouded feelings on getting back into exercising and dieting. I find that being dedicated and making small changes in my once-lethargic lifestyle opened the door to huge success, in both professional and family settings. This is a program I recommend to anyone looking to form good habits or start anew."

PEP TALK

I feel you smiling, dear Swinger! I know you're ready, I know you're pumped, I know you're excited to take this on, and that is exactly what you're going to do! I know your energy can shift day to day, so keep your foundational drive for a healthier, happier you within reach. This program is designed to let you be part of the decisions in your daily life and to let you feel your way through each week. Use accountability partners, too. No matter if your day swings into a high or low, keep your energy steady, strong, and connected. Play the middle, eliminating all the extra white noise, and you'll allow space to discover new things about yourself—an extremely empowering experience. Not only will you find a much slimmer, tighter you, but you are also going to find your strength, your ability to truly commit, and an independence that has been there all along.

CHAPTER 7

THE REBEL

YOUR PERSONALITY SNAPSHOT

> Spontaneous and impulsive

> High energy

> Live for the moment

> Not detail-oriented

> Dislike routine and complexity

> Somewhat disorganized and chaotic in planning, but effective nonetheless

> Inconsistent in dieting, exercise, and other aspects of fitness and health

> Unaware of how day-to-day decisions can affect health

> Noncommittal and often tardy

What I love about you is your live-in-the-moment zest for life! You're intensely curious, creative, optimistic, energetic, and spontaneous, thriving in a free-form approach toward life.

You're a risk taker and love beginning new things, but if activities get too structured you can become bored. You're at your best when your routine is varied and allows you to find your way through the day. If life were a bar, you'd be a pub crawl, my friend!

You're always in motion, juggling many tasks at once, without finishing all of them. Often you grind out 80 percent of a project extremely well but then stall with the remaining 20 percent. When you do complete something, however, it's right on the deadline or at the ring of the bell. In shared spaces, you frequently run late and are wishy-washy on firm commitments, but you're easily forgiven because you're so overwhelmingly well-liked. The fact that you can multitask with the best of 'em when you do arrive or commit makes up for all this.

Although your path to accomplishment is not linear, you have components that allow you to be as effective as an Organized Doer. In your mind and proven life experience, there are many ways to achieve a goal, and you're not opposed to venturing onto multiple roads to get there. Your functional chaos is what allows you to do things *your way*, and quite successfully.

You welcome sudden challenges, spur-of-the-moment events, and change. Hundreds of years ago the Greek philosopher Heraclitus, stated: "The only thing that is constant is change." This is as true now as it was then, making your openness and adaptability two of your greatest assets. Whatever change occurs, whether in the gym switching from station to station or in life's unpredictability, you are all in. Sure, you tend to be a bit disorganized, but that's okay. . . . In the game of life, your strategy is constantly changing, and that keeps you winning.

Let's drill down to some specifics and watch you in action on the job. You definitely don't get hung up on the little things. They often pass right over your head. In your mind, if they really are that important, they'll circle back and you can decide on an action then.

When it comes to team projects, you are happy to be a workhorse, executing directives. But you are happy stepping up if the team needs a leader. Additionally, when a solution is found, you're not too concerned about who gets the credit; you're just happy that your team has achieved one.

You can switch gears in an instant. No matter the change of direction or how many times it changes, you rally and put your momentum behind it. If your boss asks you to design a house, then says, "No, wait. Design a skyscraper," you're on it immediately.

This personality type is very MacGyver-esque, taking random things, thoughts, or people and establishing progress and solutions.

If I rode with you to a meeting, I'd see that your car is packed and a bit messy. And to your co-workers, your office may look just as chaotic, too, with items arranged in haphazard order, but to you this is not a problem. You're aware that it will take a few minutes to find what you're looking for when you need it, but you take the time because you know it's there.

Outside work, you are just as spontaneous and charmingly chaotic. Plan for the weekend? Forget it. You keep your days open and don't schedule the weekend until you're approaching Friday. Heck, you might throw a party at the last minute because you feel like it.

If you're a parent, you're flexible with your kids but no less attentive to their needs, even if that means the housework never fully gets done. You know they require some structure, and you provide it, while leaving room for spontaneous acts to keep it interesting, like heading out for ice cream even though it's past their bedtime. Creating experiences and connecting with your loved ones and friends takes priority over proper timing and to-do lists.

You get a kick out of seeing your kids run in different directions and just having fun. There's no one way to be a great parent.

As for relationships, either dating or marriage, you're turned on by a confident partner who allows you room to breathe and the freedom to live! A perfect date night is one that is unplanned with a "make it up as we go" mentality. You want your mate to liven things up, make you laugh, and gently smile at your disorganized way of being in the world.

Whether it's with a date, friends, or loved ones, you enjoy trying something new at restaurants. Eating is an adventure, so you love to try offbeat restaurants. Ecuadorian cuisine, anyone? The weirder the menu, the better. Ironically, you don't even need to like the food to enjoy the experience.

Often you don't know what's in your fridge but can pull something together regardless. You might even be a little kitchen phobic and not sure what to do with food—an uncertainty that makes you anxious. For this reason, you are happy to take on direction toward what to eat, as long as you're not prompted to eat the same dish at the same time every day. That's because restriction is your enemy, so stereotypical diet plans are not for you. You'll do best on an eating plan that incorporates an à la carte style of eating without too many calorie-dense ingredients and is infused with flexibility.

As for grocery shopping, you're a bit carefree with money and don't pay much attention to price and value. Nor do you rely on budgeting when you shop. You often buy items you hadn't planned on (like a random box of cookies or chips) or don't need.

A REBEL IN REAL LIFE: KELSEY

My ability to discern a Rebel's diet personality type was formed during my college years at the University of Kansas when I roomed with Kelsey, a close friend, training partner, and Division I athlete like me. She was a rower and I was a hammer thrower—that's pretty much where the similarities ended. Living together, I could see that Kelsey and I were at the opposite poles of personality, as she was the quintessential Rebel.

We both had early-morning training sessions, but whereas I would lay out every item of clothing the night before, from my sports bra to my shoes, already untied and ready for wearing, Kelsey would stumble around in the dark morning hours, trying to suit up minutes before she had to leave for practice. She'd emerge a bit tousled but dressed nonetheless with a lopsided ponytail, compared with my perfect top bun. (I was a gymnast for ten years—I couldn't help it!)

As for our normal daily routine: once we returned from practice, we'd fix breakfast. I was in charge of cooking the eggs, dicing the vegetables and avocado, and building out a fully balanced scramble, while Kelsey opened canned fruit, cut up an apple, or, her favorite, took toast duty.

She had her own style: she wore cool T-shirts and shades, every hat looked good on her, she never shied from bright colors, and she always borrowed random jewelry from my stash.

She was often past due for a manicure or pedicure with little nicks and chips, rocking flip-flops nonetheless, but she was everyone's favorite nail salon buddy because she was always down to go, gab, and have fun. She was a breath of fresh air in everyone's day—even for the manicurist.

After Kelsey went grocery shopping, I'd find some of the bags on the floor, some on the counter—half put away, half still in the bags.

It was a riot to watch her cook her meals: always loosely focused, having fun, and jamming out to music. She used few ingredients and simple recipes, but nothing was limited about her serving sizes. It was with love that she would overload my plate—more than what I'd normally eat, but we enjoyed every bite till our plates were clean. Instead of a cup or two of pasta, my plate would overflow with it. Instead of a quarter of an avocado on toast, she'd double up to two slices and use the whole thing.

I was fairly focused with my diet, even back then. But while Kelsey began each day with good intentions, she had trouble seeing the volume of what she was eating. Her portion size would vary greatly because she simply didn't give it much thought. If she saw something she wanted, she would enjoy it.

Her eating style was unpredictable—sometimes she'd nosh throughout the day and other times she'd eat three square meals. Time didn't play a role, and again, neither did portions. So easygoing and relaxed, she was down for whatever food was present.

As for working out, Kelsey was up for anything, and once she committed to an activity she was dialed in. She never slowed down, never quit, and never listened to her head telling her to stop, no matter how tired she was. She showed me what determination was, and she was the essence of willpower. She proved to me that you can live a life of extremes and still be very successful.

THE SUPPORT YOU NEED TO SUCCEED

You can reduce the chaos in your life through a little more routine, accessible patterns, a more relaxed focus, and better habits—as long as they don't get in the way of your spontaneous nature. Your energy and momentum are to be celebrated.

My diet for you involves a little nutritional babysitting, but certainly not hand holding. You'll have daily minimums for your meals, with nutrition benchmarks, not only in content but in plate volume. As for workouts, I'll hold you to a much looser schedule with baseline expectations and restrictions built within it so you can maintain that degree of freedom on which you thrive.

Ultimately, you'll feel positively reinforced at every step along the way, no matter how big or small that step is. You'll feel great about the way you look and will love your increased energy level, your improved gym skills, and even the fact that you are meeting your weekly workout minimum.

BEHAVIOR THAT ENCOURAGES WEIGHT GAIN

- Taking on too much too fast
- Skipping meals
- Overcommitting, which leads to flaking, which leads to a negative spiral
- Unconscious food portions
- Sumo-wrestler eating (one big meal a day)
- Too many liquid calories

BEHAVIOR THAT ENCOURAGES WEIGHT LOSS

- Elevated portion awareness
- One-day prepping/six-day cranking
- Gentle yet clear benchmarks
- Taking zero days off—keeping that gym bag in the car!
- Packing an emergency snack stash—having a healthy snack to reach for at all times
- Limiting perishables
- Setting up reminder alarms on your phone

THE REBEL MEAL PLAN

Your plan is all about guidelines without containment. Essentially, I'm having you go bowling in the bumper lanes, and yup—you guessed it—I'm the bumpers. I want you moving freely within your day with no expectation about time or place but equipped with the information you need to execute each meal with simplicity and ease.

Lack of portion control is a trouble spot for you; you tend to eat beyond the point of fullness as a result. I will counter that issue by volumizing your foods and eliminating empty calories that fail to fill you up. For example, instead of spending 100 calories on twenty-three M&Ms or 1/4 cup raisins, you'll enjoy 2 1/4 cups strawberries.

Understand that foods such as fruits as veggies are the most filling, with protein coming in second and fats a distant last place. Filling on the inside and slimming on the outside is a win-win.

Initially, I'll elevate your carbohydrates, then reduce them as the weeks pass. This systematic "lowering" of carbs will ramp up fat burning, which is a more effective way to drop body fat than just cutting calories. In a four-month study, British researchers discovered that dieters following occasional carb restriction lost an average of nine pounds of fat compared with five pounds lost by those following a standard calorie-restricted diet.

And you won't feel hungry with these cuts. While cutting back on your carbs, I'll increase your protein intake and stabilize your fat and water consumption.

I also want to raise your awareness of how you're feeling in order to shift you away from an "always time to eat" mentality. If you're hungry . . . eat. Thirsty . . . drink. Tired . . . sleep. Along with the focus of making you leaner during these four weeks, I want you working on staying connected to yourself and eating consciously.

Also, pay attention to the timing of your cravings and from where they originate. I'm willing to bet that your cravings are born out of inconsistent self-care when it comes to nourishment and rest. By creating stability in your life over these four weeks, you'll see a clear diminishment in your cravings.

JEN'S POWER 5 FOR REBELS

1. Use my by-the-numbers approach to meal planning, a simple format that will create stability in your health and food choices while honoring your free-form lifestyle. You'll eat five meals a day, consisting of some combination of proteins, carbs, fats, vegetables, and water. Week by week, look for progressions in your servings. This will set you up for increased metabolism.

2. Become a student of your portions, familiarizing yourself with serving sizes for each food group, and then *sticking*

with them. Examples are shown after the meal templates that follow.

3. Increase your awareness of hunger levels throughout the day. This will keep you better connected to meal timing, prevent energy dips, and keep you from reaching for empty-calorie snacks and overeating at your main meals.

   Do not skip meals, especially breakfast. Judging by the research, breakfast eaters are not only leaner than breakfast-skippers but they also have better-quality diets overall.

4. Follow the water-drinking schedule outlined in this chapter. Staying hydrated will keep everything moving through your system. You may perk up your water with a little lemon juice or sliced cucumber, and even sparkling water. Also, feel free to have coffee or tea with your meals.

5. Keep a gym bag with a change of workout clothes in your car at all times. With your spontaneity, having a workout as an option when the window presents itself will keep you in the gym on a more consistent basis.

PLANNING YOUR MEALS USING THE TEMPLATES AND SERVING SIZES

Here I show you how to put all these tools together to create your meals. Let's suppose you're in Week 3, and you want to create Meal 3 that week. You'll look through the template and see that Meal 3 is designed like this:

	Protein	Carbs	Fat	Vegetables	Water
Meal 3 (Week 3):	2	1	0	2	2

You're going to have 2 servings of protein, 1 serving of carbohydrate, 0 servings of fat, 2 servings of vegetables, and 2 servings of water.

Next, you select your servings from each nutrient group. Thus, your Meal 3 might look like this:

MEAL 3 (WEEK 3)
    2 servings of protein = 6 ounces 90% lean ground beef
    1 serving of carbohydrate = $1/2$ cup cooked brown rice
    0 servings of fat = 0
    2 servings of vegetables = 1 cup steamed broccoli and $1/2$ tomato
      (sliced)
    2 servings of water = 16 ounces water (2 cups)

Voilà—you've just created a meal following a few very simple guidelines, and you will do this for every single meal over the four-week plan.

THE MEAL PLANNING TEMPLATES FOR REBELS

Here's the overall breakdown for each week, spacing the meals $2^1/2$ to 3 hours apart. Now let's get to it!

Meal template: Protein—Carbs—Fat—Vegetables—Water

WEEK 1

	Protein	Carbs	Fat	Vegetables	Water
Meal 1:	2	2	0	0	1
Meal 2:	0	1	0	0	1
Meal 3:	1	2	0	1	1
Meal 4:	0	0	1	0	1
Meal 5:	2	0	1	1	1

WEEK 2

	Protein	Carbs	Fat	Vegetables	Water
Meal 1:	2	1	0	1	1
Meal 2:	0	1	0	0	2
Meal 3:	2	2	0	1	1
Meal 4:	0	0	1	0	2
Meal 5:	2	0	1	1	2

WEEK 3

	Protein	Carbs	Fat	Vegetables	Water
Meal 1:	3	1	0	1	1
Meal 2:	0	2	0	0	2
Meal 3:	2	1	0	2	2
Meal 4:	0	0	1	1	2
Meal 5:	2	0	1	2	2

WEEK 4

	Protein	Carbs	Fat	Vegetables	Water
Meal 1:	3	1	0	2	2
Meal 2:	0	1	0	0	2
Meal 3:	2	1	0	2	2
Meal 4:	0	0	1	1	2
Meal 5:	2	0	1	3	2

EXAMPLE DAY FOR WEEK 3

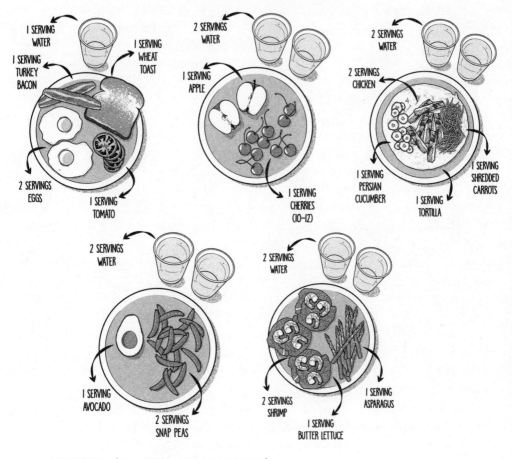

1 SERVING WATER
1 SERVING WHEAT TOAST
1 SERVING TURKEY BACON
2 SERVINGS EGGS
1 SERVING TOMATO

2 SERVINGS WATER
1 SERVING APPLE
1 SERVING CHERRIES (10–12)

2 SERVINGS WATER
2 SERVINGS CHICKEN
1 SERVING PERSIAN CUCUMBER
1 SERVING TORTILLA
1 SERVING SHREDDED CARROTS

2 SERVINGS WATER
1 SERVING AVOCADO
2 SERVINGS SNAP PEAS

2 SERVINGS WATER
2 SERVINGS SHRIMP
1 SERVING BUTTER LETTUCE
1 SERVING ASPARAGUS

PROTEIN (ALL REFLECT 1 SERVING)

BREAKFAST PROTEIN

1 large egg

3 large egg whites

3 1/2 ounces 2% Greek yogurt

1/2 cup 2% milk

2 ounces turkey sausage or bacon

1/2 ounce (2 slices) bacon

SEAFOOD PROTEIN

3 ounces salmon or halibut fillet

4 ounces whitefish, swordfish, tuna steak, or tilapia

4 ounces shrimp or scallops

1 (3-ounce) can tuna (water packed)

MEAT PROTEIN

3 ounces 90% lean ground beef

3 ounces filet mignon

3 ounces skirt steak

3 ounces loin cuts (which tend to be lean)

2 slices reduced-fat lunch meats (organic is ideal)

POULTRY PROTEIN

4 ounces white meat chicken, skin removed

3 ounces dark meat chicken, skin removed

3 ounces turkey meat, skin removed

3 ounces 93% lean ground turkey

VEGETARIAN/VEGAN PROTEIN

2 to 3 tablespoons algae (clorella/spirulina)

1 1/2 cups artichokes

1 cup black-eyed peas

1 1/2 cups green peas

1 cup edamame

1 cup tempeh

1 cup tofu

3/4 cup black beans

3/4 cup lentils

3 tablespoons hemp seeds

1/2 cup pumpkin seeds

2 cups spinach

OTHER PROTEINS

1 cup nondairy milk (almond, coconut, hemp, rice, or soy)

1/2 cup cottage cheese

1/2 cup ricotta cheese

1 to 1 1/2 scoops protein powder (whey, pea, hemp, and nondairy are all acceptable)

CARBOHYDRATES (ALL REFLECT 1 SERVING)

GRAIN-BASED CARBOHYDRATES

1/2 cup oatmeal (Jen's specs: contains 5 grams or more of fiber and under 10 grams of sugar per cooked serving)

1/2 cup oat bran

1/4 cup granola (Jen's specs: contains 5 grams or more of fiber and under 10 grams of sugar per serving)

1 cup high-fiber cereal (such as All-Bran or Fiber One)

1 slice sprouted bread

1 slice whole-wheat bread

1/2 cup brown rice or brown rice pasta

1/2 cup quinoa or quinoa pasta

1/2 cup barley

1/2 cup bulgur wheat

1 tortilla (see Jen's specs, page 225)

VEGETABLE CARBOHYDRATES

1/2 cup legumes (black beans, chickpeas, edamame, kidney beans, or lentils)

1 1/2 cups lentil soup

1 cup sweet potato or yam

FRUIT CARBOHYDRATES

1 medium apple

1/4 cup dried apricots

1 medium banana

2 cups fresh berries (strawberries, raspberries, blueberries, or blackberries)

1/2 cantaloupe

1 cup cherries

1/2 grapefruit

1 cup grapes

2 kiwi

1 nectarine

1 orange

1 peach

1 medium pear

1 cup pineapple chunks (no syrup added)

2 plums

1/2 cup stewed pitted prunes

1 tangerine

1 cup watermelon chunks

FATS (ALL REFLECT 1 SERVING)

1 ounce almonds (23)

1 ounce cashews (16 to 18)

1 ounce pecans (20 halves)

1 ounce pistachios (49)

1 ounce walnuts (12 to 14 halves)

2 tablespoons almond butter

2 tablespoons peanut butter

1 1/2 ounces natural, hard cheese (Cheddar,

mozzarella, Swiss, or Parmesan)

1/2 cup hummus

1/2 avocado

1 ounce pine nuts, not oiled

1 ounce sunflower seeds, not oiled

1 ounce flaxseed

1 tablespoon olive oil, coconut oil, canola oil, or flaxseed oil

2 teaspoons butter

2 teaspoons margarine,
    trans-fat free

1 tablespoon mayonnaise

2 tablespoons reduced-fat or
    light mayonnaise

1 tablespoon salad dressing

2 tablespoons reduced-fat or
    low-calorie salad dressing

VEGETABLES (ALL REFLECT 1 SERVING)

2 cups alfalfa sprouts

3 cups arugula

2 cups asparagus

2 cups bell pepper

2 cups bok choy

2 cups broccoli

2 cups Brussels sprouts

2 cups shredded cabbage

1 cup carrots

2 cups cauliflower

2 cups cauliflower rice

2 cups celery

3 cups collard greens

2 cups cucumber

2 cups eggplant

2 cups endive

2 cups green beans

$1/2$ cup green onions (scallions)

$1/2$ cup jalapeño or other hot
    pepper

3 cups fresh kale

1 cup leeks

3 cups lettuce (all varieties)

1 cup mushrooms

1 cup onion

1 cup parsley

1 cup radishes

2 cups snap peas

3 cups fresh spinach

$1^1/2$ cups squash (all varieties)

1 cup Swiss chard

$1/2$ tomato

3 cups turnip greens

1 cup wax beans

$1^1/2$ cups zucchini

Water

1 serving of water = 8 ounces
    (1 cup)

Meet Kiran

"Jen is truly one of a kind. She has been an inspiration to me in more ways than one, but she started off as my trainer. I run a business where my doors are open twenty-four hours a day, so every hour is nonstop. I rarely plan anything because I never know what's going to happen next and no two days are the same. Because of this I've always

Enhancing the flavors of your food is key to not only enjoying them but sustaining these healthy meal combinations in your diet plan. The following is what I call your "Yum-Yum List," because these are all Jen-approved items that will make each bite more delicious than the last *without* compromising your progress on your waistline.

Basic Seasonings

Salt

Black pepper

Lemon pepper

Red pepper flakes

Chili powder

Garlic powder

Onion powder

Cumin

Paprika (regular or smoked)

Turmeric

Herbs—Dried or Fresh

Basil

Chives

Cilantro

Dill

Garlic

Oregano

Parsley

Rosemary

Sage

Thyme

Condiments

Ketchup—limited

Mustard (all kinds)

Mayonnaise—limited

Hummus

Barbecue sauce—limited

Hot sauce (all kinds)

Miscellaneous

Pickles

Lemon

Lime

Apple cider vinegar

Balsamic vinegar

Coconut oil

Olive oil

Soy sauce

Chia seeds

Hemp seeds

Agave

Honey

Cooking spray (vegetable, coconut, or olive oil)

struggled to follow any kind of diet plan. Jen's program has given me the freedom to choose in the moment based on what I have access to, and because of the guidelines she has set, I *know* I am making the right choices. I cannot say enough how much stress this has alleviated in my life. My health and fitness are a huge priority for me, so knowing that I can still have a plan that is just as on-the-fly as my hectic business schedule and chaotic lifestyle has made all the difference. Jen clearly understood my personal needs and schedule, and for the first time I felt like I was on a diet that I could live on!

"As a trainer, she has a unique ability to connect with people to understand their strengths and weaknesses, both physically and emotionally. She is the most engaged person I've ever met. She has motivated me on my toughest days, has been there for me during my proudest moments, and continues to remind me of the importance of decision making.

"Ultimately, it's the choices that we make that define us, and Jen has never let me forget that. She enables me to be a better version of myself in every aspect of my life. Thank you, Jen, for all the love and support and most important your unwavering friendship."

PEP TALK

You may be unpredictable, but you are extremely powerful and effective. Never forget this. On the surface, you may be bubbly and fun, but I know there's a fighter in there. Never trade in the dreamer, but when it comes to your health, give that fighter a stronger voice. You're going to be successful, and you're going to do it with ease, especially since I've allowed you so much freedom. Lean in to that open space while executing the minimums I've given you, and you will see the weight fade off. You will feel your energy climb, and you'll find yourself loving your body more than you thought possible. I look to you to be an example for the others, embracing your shape and thriving because you honor yourself better than anyone else. There are such good things ahead for you, my Rebel!

CHAPTER 8

THE EVERYDAY HERO

YOUR PERSONALITY SNAPSHOT

> Collaborative and adaptive

> Friendly and relate well to others

> Want to be respected, liked, and approved of

> Selfless and a committed friend

> Overloaded at times, by taking on too much

> Motivating and supportive of others

> Tend to put yourself lower on the priority list because you're so busy taking care of others

> Subsist on a lot of grab-and-go foods or drive-throughs and eating on the run

> Prefer to eat with others rather than alone

> Inconsistent with exercise because of time-constraint-based excuses

As a personal trainer, I can relate to you: you feel best when helping, motivating, or mentoring others. You listen with your heart and worry more about relationships and harmony, sometimes to the point of being taken advantage of. You do your best to build consensus and make sure that no one's feelings are ignored or overlooked. Put simply, you don't want to let anyone down. You're the caregiver, the super parent, the family steward, the volunteer, the best of the best friends, the go-to person in your family or group of friends, the protector, or all of the above. You have a strong personality gift called selflessness. This quality makes you great at nurturing relationships, and it practically defines you.

Your personality type, with its strong bonds and tight social connections, is good for your health. In a 2009 study published in *Perspectives in Psychological Science*, researchers found that social support leads to stronger coping skills, healthier behavior, and better adherence to medical advice from doctors and other health care professionals. Bonding with people, at which you excel, also reduces stress and improves immunity—so making friends becomes, in effect, a prescription for well-being.

In the professional world, you perform well in almost any business that involves people, as long as it's a somewhat nonconfrontational workplace. You dislike conflict. In fact, you are the "Why can't we all just get along?" person on the team or in the department. You find value in the relationships you build, and you care about how everyone feels about their work, so you make a point to give feedback and positive reinforcement. You are very likable, work well with others, and promote harmony.

You thrive in a team environment because of the human connection, and you do not work at your best alone. You prefer to lead, but are happy to follow; just put you on a team, for goodness' sake!

When you are part of a work team or department, you're the cheerleader, building team spirit and strengthening cooperation. You may have a difficult time saying no, even when you're already overloaded with work.

You are often wrapped up in causes—and very compassionate with those who may be hurting. You are patient, a good listener, and known for your integrity.

In your social media posts, you love to share inspirational messages or quotes. Even the lock screen on your smartphone enlightens you with sayings that inspire you.

Outside work, your home is warm and inviting. If you have kids, you understand the incredible role you play in their lives, and you provide the right amount of guidance and understanding, but you're the first to admit your mistakes or layers of imperfection. If the school needs someone to chaperone, run the carpool, or head up teacher appreciation week, you're among the first to volunteer.

You manage the family finances, college fund, and budget in a characteristically protective way to fulfill your primary goal of taking care of your family. Your personality type tends to take care of others and not yourself. In other words, your personal priorities often get shoved to the bottom of your to-do list.

You love to share meals with your loved ones. There's nothing better than socializing around a great meal, at your home, during family dinners, at parties with friends, or during nights out at restaurants. The enjoyment of food rests largely on whom it is being enjoyed with. Eating alone or cooking for one is dissatisfying for you, so you'll just grab some takeout instead or do a pantry dive.

You're so busy sometimes catering to others that you feel it's impossible to eat enough nourishing foods on a daily basis. You graze or nibble all day long but seldom sit down with a plate filled with balanced nutrition. You're always noshing on bars or leftovers, half-eating your meal, or eating snack packs of something. These habits often leave you hungry and vulnerable to processed fast food or grab-and-go snacks that are not particularly healthy.

You can't be bothered with paying attention to portion sizes, counting calories or points, and trying to fuel your body with healthy foods. It's so much easier to grab whatever is most accessible. Sometimes it's healthy; sometimes it's not. Either way, you just never seem to establish a routine or momentum to help you drop pounds or optimize your health. Put simply, you just don't give a #&@$!

You tolerate being hungry to the extreme, but your stomach grumbling creates anxiety because you know you need a healthy option but you feel stuck on how to make that happen in the moment. Ultimately, you always feel a sense of despair. Even *if* you could get your hands on a healthy snack today, you question how likely it would be for you to have one the next day and then the next, until you arrive at the feeling of "This is too hard to keep up," and you quit before you start. Despite this and the fact that you may be overweight, the idea of missing a meal is stressful. Your hunger for recognition tends to translate into cravings and comfort food.

Because your own needs tend to be ignored, fitting in exercise can be a challenge. Unlike other personality types, you know exactly how to be successful in your fitness journey and have experienced it multiple times. With Everyday Heroes, it's not as much about educating yourself or knowing what to do to get healthy, but about doing it! Time and again, you make concessions when it comes to your weight-loss and wellness goals and allow your workout program to taper off because life intervenes. Your excuse is often that you don't have enough time. If you happen to carve out a little time for yourself, all you really want to do is sit and rest because you feel so low in energy. Even the thought of training makes you tired. Since something's got to give, you always choose to give up your workout.

Deep down, you know that a healthy body is an active body, and being healthy bolsters your ability to care for others. So when you fall short, you feel ashamed and put yourself down for not being consistent. That's the interior "you"; the exterior puts on an "I'm fine" front. You want people to see you as having it all together, all the time. Supportive, loyal, and dependable, you often need people to motivate you to exercise and to keep you engaged in a diet and exercise routine.

AN EVERYDAY HERO IN REAL LIFE: CINDY

Right after another stretch of family holidays, Cindy saw a glimpse of herself in a Facebook album posted by her sister. She was caught off guard: "Is that really me?"

"I looked dumpy, older than my age, and run-down," she said. "That was when I realized that I needed to make some changes." I began working with Cindy shortly thereafter.

I suggested that she also recruit her husband to get on board at home. He wanted to lose weight, too, and Cindy's success would hinge partly on his support. I know the research on the importance of family support. Many studies demonstrate that a change in your partner's health behavior is often associated with a change in your behavior.

Research published in 2015 in the *European Journal of Nutrition* found that if male and female partners/spouses went on a diet together and/or an exercise program, both would lose weight and be more successful than if they did these things on their own. Men and women are more likely to make a positive health behavior change if their partner does, too, and with a stronger effect than if the partner had been consistently healthy in that domain. So I was glad Cindy was open to including her husband.

I designed a diet that would fit her maxed-out lifestyle. The focus was looking ahead in the week to meet each complicated day with a simple food formula. We planned a week's worth of dinners so we could shop for the ingredients on the weekend before as well as stock up on nutritious foods that she could grab at a moment's notice. She kept water and healthy snacks, such as fruit and almonds, with her at all times so she would never find herself in a position where a low-nutrient, fattening food was her only option. The whole point of the plan was to set her up for success while getting out of her default mode to strengthen her power of choice.

Cindy saw immediate results. She noticed she had more energy, and her sensations of hunger returned (yay for metabolism!). As a chronic headache sufferer, she had experienced only one in the time since we began our program. Cindy lost twelve pounds in the first month. Her stamina in workouts had doubled. Her too-tight jeans were getting loose. And she was looking more shapely than she had in a long time.

Cindy was a joy to train because she cared about the quality of her work. She wanted to make it clear to me that she was committed, so she was very communicative and worked out hard. She'd often come in late, frazzled as always but unfazed by it. She gave me all she had when she got there, though.

Cindy never wanted to know the "whys" behind the workout; she preferred to just have me put her through her paces. Sometimes, though, she'd feel frustrated, probably conflicted over her shifting priorities. It wasn't often, but there were times when she teared up with questions that overwhelmed her: "Can I really keep this up? How can I do this another day, let alone a whole week, or the rest of the year? Will I ever not feel so tired? Will I ever hit my goal?"

Cindy could get pretty tough on herself to the point of feeling guilty about taking so much time for herself, especially when her progress was hinging on her ability to be consistent. Ironically, she carried guilt through the sessions because she felt she was constantly underperforming. This was the source of her personal stress; she felt like she was a failure, whether she was investing in herself or not.

Just as important as moving her body was to her weight-loss routine, we had to build dialogue around what I call "an inside job." I explained to her that self-talk must look at facts and truths before automatic condemnations take over. For example, we were running, and she kept needing to stop. This frustrated and angered her: "I've made all this effort to be so consistent in training with you, so this shouldn't be so hard."

Inside job: "I was up with my sick child all night, so I barely slept. I didn't eat breakfast, because I forgot about it and left it on the kitchen counter." Reality check: "No food and no sleep has affected me in a big way. Therefore, this is simply where my body and energy are *today* and not a reflection of the last month of work or my ability to reach my goals. I'm giving the best I have each day, and that will always be enough."

I'd remind her that making time for herself, whether it be for physical or emotional reprieve, would ultimately be the best gift she could give her family and loved ones. After all, how could she go through her day as the woman that she loved being if she was too broken down to do so. This realization always brought her through her slump and she'd crank in her workouts, focused, intentional, and full of desire.

Eventually, movement became an anchor for her. She loved it because of the way it made her feel and also the way it helped her stick to her diet. She knew that one bad meal choice would erase that workout, and she wasn't willing to give that up.

After many consistent weeks in the gym, exercise became much easier, and I could see the sense of accomplishment on her face. In turn, she could then increase her intensity. She was stronger and had more momentum. For her to keep it up, she needed to remember where she started and remind herself that the days of putting herself last on the list were over.

I loved training her. It never ceased to amaze me how caring she was. She always invited me to her family gatherings. She would give me the perfect gifts, because she truly listened to me, investing in who I was. There were days I would joke that instead of her writing me checks for training, I should be writing her checks for therapy.

After about six months, I saw a different woman. Cindy had a 40-pound weight loss, and she reached her goal weight of 125 pounds a year later. Her overall stamina in her training was as impressive as her weight loss. Her conditioning, her strength, and her mental edge were all dialed in.

What about her husband? He was successful, too: a sixty-pound weight loss in that same year. With their newfound fitness and health habits, both Cindy and her husband became even stronger role models for their kids.

THE SUPPORT YOU NEED TO SUCCEED

The Everyday Hero definitely needs a support team—in the gym and in the kitchen—to stay on track. But the real key to success is to actually ask your support team for help, so you can ultimately invest more time in yourself. It's okay to do this, although I know you may be reluctant. Just do it gradually.

As the only female trainer on *The Biggest Loser*, I felt like I had to be the strong one. I was reluctant at first to accept support from my contestants, but I quickly learned how powerful their support for me was. From their handwritten letters to making sure that I was taking as good of care of myself as I was them, I learned how showing my own need for support really brought us closer. I didn't realize how much I needed their help—and most important, to give myself the permission to receive it. When you need help and support, and I assure you it's there, don't be afraid to embrace it.

I will prove to you that the world won't end if you have to ask for support—but your life will actually get better! When you rely a little more on others, your baseline health will improve. You'll get more sleep, focus on staying hydrated, and be more nourished. In short, forget your fears about asking for help! You'll find that people in your life want to help and give back to you. You deserve to have your personal health needs met just as much as everyone else.

BEHAVIOR THAT ENCOURAGES WEIGHT GAIN
- Negative self-talk
- Being a martyr and making excuses
- Long periods of time with no food

- Lack of sleep
- High stress
- Taking on everything by yourself

BEHAVIOR THAT ENCOURAGES WEIGHT LOSS

- Setting aside time for yourself (Daily 10: ten minutes to begin, end, and/or reset your day)
- Not quitting before month two!
- Self-care (for example, investing in your appearance, having regular health checkups, and getting more rest)
- Packing-up/prepping each morning for the day
- Consistency in workouts
- Meditation and breathing exercises
- Yoga

THE EVERYDAY HERO MEAL PLAN

You've proven time and again that there is nothing out of your reach when you set your mind to it—including losing weight and getting in shape. This is your truth, and it's why so many people count on you. Well, for the first time, your weight-loss and wellness journey will be applied to the foolproof formula of *you*.

I designed this to be a very replicable plan that will not compete with the rest of your busy day, as no real cooking is required, with the exception of your final meal at dinner. And many of those dinners let you use your trusty, time-saving slow cooker.

Because you tend to not eat enough, this plan meets your needs for baseline nutrition. As a result, you'll quickly feel your body begin to reboot with greater energy, thanks to the nutritional benchmarks I've set for you each day. Nourishing grab-and-go meals will be your anchor, and although snacking is programmed for you in each day, you're strictly prohibited from using snacks as a replacement for a meal. I know this can feel like a firm request at first, but when you eat more real produce and fewer "drinkable" and shelf-stable "ready-to-eat" packaged meals, you'll quickly see a shift in your physique and in your energy.

As an Everyday Hero, you thrive on being there for others. But how far will you let things go in your health and, consequently, your happiness before you're willing to make a change? Let me step up for you and invest in your life by teaching you how to invest in it yourself. My greatest concern for you, my dear Hero, is that because of your resilience, you take a long time to break down, agreeing to compromise after compromise, so when you do break down, you break hard. The program I've developed here is my sincere investment in you. It will preserve your independence and improve your strengths. Accept my support and belief in you, and let's take this first step together.

JEN'S POWER 5 FOR EVERYDAY HEROES

1. Invest in yourself the way you invest in others. This isn't the easiest task for Everyday Heroes, but when you do it, you will thrive. Begin in small ways like buying workout gear that you feel good in, taking just ten minutes of uninterrupted quiet time for yourself to slow down, or even giving yourself permission to say no when there is something else that may better serve you.

2. For many breakfasts and lunches, all you have to do is whip up one of my nutritious shakes. They remove all obstacles for you when it comes to getting nutrition consistently—a key factor in weight loss—which is why I created them just for you. They, along with all the recipes I'll share with you, require little planning so you can keep losing weight—and quickly.

3. Plan your workouts for the week at the *beginning* of each week. When you hold time aside in advance for an activity, you are much more likely to do it.

4. Set yourself up for success by never missing a meal prep day. Having your bakes ready, snacks prepared, and healthy ingredients on hand will ensure your success in this plan. If you don't get enough calories in, your body won't drop

the weight—so prepping your meals and hitting your "watermarks" will be game changers for you.

5. Talk to the people in your life about what you're taking on. A lot of your happiness is based on knowing you can be there for the ones you care about; it's time to allow them to be there for you as well. This support and acknowledgment from them is just what you need to give yourself the okay and truly take on this transformation.

WEEK 1

Week 1 Grocery List

(Many of these ingredients you will use again in future weeks.)

PROTEIN

6 large eggs

5 boneless skinless chicken breasts

4 ounces sliced white-meat chicken or turkey

1 pound 93% lean ground turkey

8 ounces 90% lean ground beef

PRODUCE

1 avocado

2 bananas

1 small package blueberries

2 cups strawberries

1 lemon

1 lime

1 pear

1 small bunch of basil

4 bell peppers (any color)

1 cup Brussels sprouts

1 (10-ounce) package shredded carrots

1 bunch cilantro

1 head garlic

5 cups fresh kale

8 ounces cremini mushrooms

1 red onion

2 yellow onions

5 ounces fresh spinach

1 large tomato

2 to 3 cups veggies for *DIY Stir-Fry (page 254)* (broccoli, peppers, onions, etc.)

5 ounces sweet potato

DAIRY

1 individual portion 2% Greek yogurt

1 package sliced cheese

1 (16-ounce) container cottage cheese

1 (8-ounce) package shredded mozzarella cheese

STARCHES

1 medium container (18 ounces) old-fashioned oats

1 loaf sprouted bread

1 (15-ounce) package quinoa

1 (32-ounce) package brown rice

NUTS/OILS

1 bottle olive oil

1 small package pine nuts

SPICES/CONDIMENTS

Salt

Pepper

Red pepper flakes

Chili powder

Garlic powder

Cumin

Dried oregano

Smoked paprika

Tomato paste

Honey or agave

OTHER

32 ounces unsweetened vanilla almond milk

1 medium jar almond or peanut butter

1 (8-ounce) package unsweetened coconut flakes

1 small jar jam (any flavor)

1 small package chia seeds

1 small packed hemp seeds

1 jar of your favorite salsa

1 packet taco seasoning

1 (15-ounce) can black beans

1 (14 1/2-ounce) can diced tomatoes

1 (28-ounce) can crushed tomatoes

32 ounces chicken stock

Hot sauce (optional)

Low-sodium soy sauce (optional)

1 small bottle vanilla extract

1 (10-ounce) package dark chocolate chips

1 container protein powder (2 pounds net weight)

1 can cooking spray (vegetable, coconut, or olive oil)

Prepare

6 servings *No-Bake Bites*
(*page 205*)

2 servings *Burger Bake*
(*page 250*)

Note: For your *Burger Bake (page 250),* you will completely set up the dish without actually cooking it today. Prep it in the baking dish, place a lid on it, and refrigerate. The nights these are on your plan, all you need to do is take the lid off, throw them in the oven, and enjoy!

Snack Stash: This week, your daily snack is two mini energy balls called *No-Bake Bites (page 205).* Pack them with you every day, as they *must* be consumed within each day outside a regular meal. They come in handy when you need to grab some instant nutrition and fight cravings.

MONDAY

BREAKFAST
Simple Shake #1 (page 222)
Watermark: Hit 25 ounces water anytime before lunch

LUNCH
Open-Faced Sandwich

Layer 1 slice Cheddar or mozzarella, 1 cup fresh spinach, 4 ounces sliced lean white meat (turkey or chicken), and 1/2 tomato, sliced (optional), on top of 1 slice sprouted bread
Watermark: Hit 40 ounces water

DINNER
Slow Cooker Shredded Chicken 1.0 (page 280) (over 1 cup brown rice)
Watermark: Hit 50 ounces water (60 minutes before bedtime)

TUESDAY

BREAKFAST
1 cup 2% Greek yogurt with 1 cup fresh blueberries and 1 1/2 teaspoons honey or agave
Watermark: Hit 25 ounces water

LUNCH
Simple Shake #2 (page 222)
Watermark: Hit 40 ounces water

DINNER
Burger Bake (page 250)
Watermark: Hit 50 ounces water (60 minutes before bedtime)

WEDNESDAY

BREAKFAST
Simple Shake #1 (page 222)
Watermark: Hit 25 ounces water

LUNCH
Open-Faced Sandwich
Layer 1 slice Cheddar or mozzarella, 1 cup fresh spinach,
4 ounces sliced lean white meat (turkey or chicken), and
1/2 tomato, sliced (optional), on top of 1 slice sprouted bread
Watermark: Hit 40 ounces water

DINNER
Spinach and Pear Salad (page 239)
Watermark: Hit 50 ounces water (60 minutes before bedtime)

THURSDAY

BREAKFAST
1 cup 2% Greek yogurt with 1 cup fresh blueberries and
1^1/$_2$ teaspoons honey or agave
Watermark: Hit 25 ounces water

LUNCH
Simple Shake #2 (page 222)
Watermark: Hit 40 ounces water

DINNER
Burger Bake (page 250)
Watermark: Hit 50 ounces water (60 minutes before bedtime)

FRIDAY

Upon waking: 10 ounces water

BREAKFAST
Simple Shake #1 (page 222)
Watermark: Hit 25 ounces water

LUNCH
Open-Faced Sandwich
>Layer 1 slice Cheddar or mozzarella, 1 cup fresh spinach, 4 ounces sliced lean white meat (turkey or chicken), and 1/2 tomato, sliced (optional), on top of 1 slice sprouted bread

Watermark: Hit 40 ounces water

DINNER
One-Pot Mexican Quinoa (page 270)
Watermark: Hit 50 ounces water (60 minutes before bedtime)

SATURDAY

BREAKFAST
1 cup 2% Greek yogurt with 1 cup fresh blueberries and 1 1/2 teaspoons honey or agave syrup
Watermark: Hit 25 ounces water

LUNCH
Simple Shake #2 (page 222)
Watermark: Hit 40 ounces water

DINNER
Spicy Stuffed Peppers (page 285)
Watermark: Hit 50 ounces water (60 minutes before bedtime)

SUNDAY

Upon waking: 10 ounces water

BREAKFAST
Blended Shake 1.0 (page 217)
Watermark: Hit 25 ounces water

LUNCH
2 large eggs (cooked any style), 1 slice sprouted bread, and 2 cups strawberries

Watermark: Hit 40 ounces water

DINNER
DIY Stir-Fry (page 254) (with chicken)

Watermark: Hit 50 ounces water (60 minutes before bedtime)

WEEK 2

Week 2 Grocery List
(Many of these ingredients may be left over from Week 1. Recheck your stash before buying more.)

PROTEIN
- 15 large eggs
- 2 boneless skinless chicken breasts
- 2 pounds 93% lean ground turkey
- 6 ounces flank steak
- 6 ounces whitefish
- 3 (5-ounce) cans tuna (water packed)

PRODUCE
- 2 Granny Smith apples
- 1 avocado
- 4 bananas
- 1 lemon
- 1 lime
- 7 pears (or similar fruit if not in season)
- 1 bunch asparagus
- 1 green bell pepper
- 1 red bell pepper
- 12-ounce package broccoli florets
- 1 small package shredded cabbage
- 1 bundle celery
- 1 ear of corn
- 1 cucumber
- 1 head garlic
- 5 ounces fresh kale
- 1 head butter lettuce (for tacos)
- 1 head romaine lettuce
- 1 bundle green onions (scallions)
- 1 yellow onion
- 10 to 15 ounces fresh spinach
- 1 summer squash
- 1 pint cherry tomatoes
- 1 medium tomato
- 1 zucchini

DAIRY

1 (8-ounce) package shredded mozzarella cheese

4 to 6 ounces grated Parmesan cheese

STARCHES

1 medium container (18 ounces) old-fashioned oats

1 (32-ounce) package brown rice

1 (15-ounce) package brown rice pasta

NUTS/OILS

1 small jar coconut oil

1 medium bottle olive oil

SPICES/CONDIMENTS

Salt

Black pepper

Chipotle pepper powder

Garlic powder

Dried basil

Dried oregano

Dried thyme

Ground cinnamon

Ground cumin

Mustard

Tomato paste

Low-sodium soy sauce

White wine vinegar

Honey

OTHER

32 ounces unsweetened vanilla almond milk

8 ounces unsweetened coconut flakes

1 small package dried fruit (your choice)

1 small package chia seeds

1 small package sesame seeds

8 ounces panko or regular bread crumbs

1 small package cornstarch

1 (15-ounce) can black beans

1 (13-ounce) jar marinara sauce

1 container protein powder (2 pounds)

1 can cooking spray (vegetable, coconut, or olive oil)

Prepare

6 hard-boiled eggs

6 *Oatmeal Muffins* (page 207)

3 servings *Tuna Salad* (page 240)

2 *Turkey Bake* (page 288)

Note: For your *Turkey Bake (page 288),* you will completely set up the dish without actually cooking it today. Prep it in the baking dish, place a lid on it, and refrigerate. The nights these are on your plan, all you need to do is take the lid off, throw them in the oven, and enjoy!

Snack Stash: This week, your daily snack is 1 pear and 1 hard-boiled egg. Pack them with you every day, as they *must* be consumed within each day outside a regular meal. They come in handy when you need to grab some instant nutrition and fight cravings.

MONDAY

BREAKFAST
Simple Shake #3 (page 223)
Watermark: Hit 25 ounces water

LUNCH
Tuna Salad (page 240) (1/3 of the recipe, on spinach)
Watermark: Hit 40 ounces water

DINNER
6 *Slow Cooker Turkey Meatballs (page 282)* (over 1 cup brown rice pasta)
Watermark: Hit 55 ounces water (60 minutes before bedtime)

TUESDAY

BREAKFAST
2 *Oatmeal Muffins (page 207)*
Watermark: Hit 25 ounces water

LUNCH
Simple Shake #4 (page 223)
Watermark: Hit 40 ounces water

DINNER
Turkey Bake (page 288)
Watermark: Hit 55 ounces water (60 minutes before bedtime)

WEDNESDAY

BREAKFAST
Simple Shake #3 (page 223)
Watermark: Hit 25 ounces water

LUNCH
Tuna Salad (page 240) (1/3 of the recipe, on spinach)
Watermark: Hit 40 ounces water

DINNER
Southwest Veggie Chop (page 238)
Watermark: Hit 55 ounces water (60 minutes before bedtime)

THURSDAY

BREAKFAST
2 Oatmeal Muffins (page 207)
Watermark: Hit 25 ounces water

LUNCH
Simple Shake #4 (page 223)
Watermark: Hit 40 ounces water

DINNER
Turkey Bake (page 288)
Watermark: Hit 55 ounces water (60 minutes before bedtime)

FRIDAY

BREAKFAST
Simple Shake #3 (page 223)
Watermark: Hit 25 ounces water

LUNCH
Tuna Salad (page 240) (1/3 of the recipe, on spinach)
Watermark: Hit 40 ounces water

DINNER
Soy-Honey Chicken with Broccoli (page 284) (over 1 cup
    brown rice)
Watermark: Hit 55 ounces water (60 minutes before bedtime)

SATURDAY

BREAKFAST
2 Oatmeal Muffins (page 207)
Watermark: Hit 25 ounces water

LUNCH
Simple Shake #4 (page 223)
Watermark: Hit 40 ounces water

DINNER
Butter Lettuce Fish Tacos with Spicy Apple Slaw (page 252)
Watermark: Hit 55 ounces water (60 minutes before bedtime)

SUNDAY

BREAKFAST
Blended Shake 1.0 (page 217)
Watermark: Hit 25 ounces water

LUNCH
Green Omelet (page 204)
Watermark: Hit 40 ounces water

DINNER
Steak and Eggs with Pan-Roasted Tomatoes (page 211)
Watermark: Hit 55 ounces water (60 minutes before bedtime)

Week 3 Grocery List

(Many of these ingredients may be left over from Weeks 1 and 2. Recheck your stash before buying more.)

PROTEIN

- 7 large eggs
- 2 boneless skinless chicken breasts
- 10 ounces ground bison
- 6 ounces cooked shrimp

PRODUCE

- 1 avocado
- 7 bananas
- 12 ounces blueberries
- 16 ounces strawberries
- 3 kiwi or peaches (or in-season fruit)
- 2 lemons
- 1 small package pomegranate seeds
- 1 bundle asparagus
- 1 small package basil
- 1 (12-ounce) package broccoli
- 8 ounces shaved Brussels sprouts
- 1 (12-ounce) package cauliflower
- 1 small bundle chives
- 1 head garlic
- 8 cups fresh baby kale
- 1 head romaine lettuce
- 1 onion
- 1 small package parsley
- 2 cups fresh spinach
- 4 medium sweet potatoes
- 1 pint cherry tomatoes

DAIRY

- 2% Greek yogurt
- 8 ounces shredded Cheddar cheese
- 4 to 6 ounces shredded Parmesan cheese

STARCHES

- 1 medium container (18 ounces) old-fashioned oats (Jen's specs: contains 5 grams or more of fiber and less than 10 grams of sugar per serving)
- 1 box granola (Jen's specs: contains 5 grams or more of fiber and less than 10 grams of sugar per serving)

1 (14- to 16-ounce) package
   black rice

1 (16-ounce) package brown
   rice pasta

1 (32-ounce) package quinoa

NUTS/OILS

16 ounces almonds

1 package almond slivers

16 ounces cashews

16 ounces pecans

1 small package pine nuts

16 ounces walnuts

1 small bottle balsamic
   vinegar

1 medium bottle olive oil

1 small bottle rice wine
   vinegar

SPICES/CONDIMENTS

Salt

Black pepper

Lemon pepper

Red pepper flakes

Chili powder

Garlic powder

Paprika

Ground cumin

Dijon mustard

Dried basil

Dried oregano

Onion powder

OTHER

Unsweetened vanilla almond
   milk

Pitted dates

Golden raisins

Chia seeds

1 (15-ounce) can black beans

1 (15-ounce) can red kidney
   beans

1 can chicken stock

1 (14-ounce) can diced
   tomatoes

1 small jar sun-dried
   tomatoes, in oil

Capers

Honey

1 can cooking spray
   (vegetable, coconut, or
   olive oil)

Prepare

6 *Egg Bakes (page 200)*

3 servings *Shaved Brussels
   Sprouts Salad (page 238)*

2 *Bison Bake (page 246)*

Note: For your *Bison Bake (page 246),* you will completely set up the dish without actually cooking it today. Prep it in the baking dish, place a lid on it, and refrigerate. The nights these are on your plan, all you need to do is take the lid off, throw them in the oven, and enjoy!

Snack Stash: This week your daily snack is 1 banana and a pre-packaged serving of almonds or pecans. Pack them with you every day, as they *must* be consumed within each day outside a regular meal. They come in handy when you need to grab some instant nutrition and fight cravings.

MONDAY

BREAKFAST
2 Egg Bakes (page 200)
1 kiwi or peach
Watermark: Hit 30 ounces water

LUNCH
Simple Shake #1 (page 222) (increase protein powder to 1½ scoops)
Watermark: Hit 50 ounces water

DINNER
Slow Cooker Sweet Potato Chili (page 282)
Watermark: Hit 65 ounces water (45 minutes before bedtime)

TUESDAY

BREAKFAST
Blended Shake 2.0 (page 217)
Watermark: Hit 30 ounces water

LUNCH
Shaved Brussels Sprouts Salad (page 238) (⅓ of the recipe)
Watermark: Hit 50 ounces water

DINNER
Bison Bake (page 246)
Watermark: Hit 65 ounces water (45 minutes before bedtime)

WEDNESDAY

BREAKFAST
2 *Egg Bakes* (*page 200*)
1 kiwi or peach
Watermark: Hit 30 ounces water

LUNCH
Simple Shake #1 (*page 222*) (increase protein powder to
1½ scoops)
Watermark: Hit 50 ounces water

DINNER
The Kale Salad (*page 232*) (with 5 ounces chicken, optional)
Watermark: Hit 65 ounces water (45 minutes before bedtime)

THURSDAY

BREAKFAST
Blended Shake 2.0 (*page 217*)
Watermark: Hit 30 ounces water

LUNCH
Shaved Brussels Sprouts Salad (*page 238*) (⅓ of the recipe)
Watermark: Hit 50 ounces water

DINNER
Bison Bake (*page 246*)
Watermark: Hit 65 ounces water (45 minutes before bedtime)

FRIDAY

BREAKFAST
2 *Egg Bakes* (*page 200*)
1 kiwi or peach
Watermark: Hit 30 ounces water

LUNCH

Simple Shake #1 (page 222) (increase protein powder to 1¹/₂ scoops)

Watermark: Hit 50 ounces water

DINNER

Shrimp Pasta (page 277)

Watermark: Hit 65 ounces water (45 minutes before bedtime)

SATURDAY

BREAKFAST

Blended Shake 2.0 (page 217)

Watermark: Hit 30 ounces water

LUNCH

Shaved Brussels Sprouts Salad (page 238) (¹/₃ of the recipe)

Watermark: Hit 50 ounces water

DINNER

One-Pot Chicken (page 269)

Watermark: Hit 65 ounces water (45 minutes before bedtime)

SUNDAY

BREAKFAST

Crunchy Oats (page 199)

Watermark: Hit 30 ounces water

LUNCH

Black Bean Egg Scramble (page 198)

Watermark: Hit 50 ounces water

DINNER

Pan-Seared Salmon with Garlicky Kale (page 272)

Watermark: Hit 65 ounces water (45 minutes before bedtime)

Week 4 Grocery List

(Many of these ingredients may be left over from Weeks 1, 2, and 3. Recheck your stash before buying more.)

PROTEIN

16 large eggs

2 boneless skinless chicken breasts

8 ounces chicken sausage

1 pound 93% lean ground turkey

6 to 8 ounces skirt steak

2 (6-ounce) salmon fillets

12 shrimp (peeled and deveined)

PRODUCE

7 apples

2 bananas

18 ounces blueberries

32 ounces strawberries

4 lemons

1 lime

1 small package pomegranate seeds

10 ounces arugula

1 small bundle asparagus

2 orange bell peppers

3 red bell peppers

4 cups Brussels sprouts

1 pound cauliflower rice (Trader Joe's has a good one, or see page 269)

1 small bunch celery

1 head garlic

1 to 2 jalapeños

5 ounces fresh baby kale

2 heads romaine lettuce

8 ounces cremini mushrooms

1 small bundle green onions (scallions)

1 red onion

2 yellow onions

5 ounces fresh spinach

2 medium sweet potatoes

1 pint cherry tomatoes

DAIRY

1/2 gallon 2% milk

16 ounces cottage cheese

8 ounces shredded mozzarella cheese

1 to 2 ounces Parmesan cheese

STARCHES

1 (14-ounce) package black rice

1 (32-ounce) package brown rice

10 to 12 ounces almond or buckwheat flour (optional)

NUTS/OILS

16 ounces cashews

16 ounces walnuts

1 medium bottle olive oil

SPICES/CONDIMENTS

Salt

Black pepper

Red pepper flakes

Garlic powder

Onion powder

Basil

Cilantro, fresh

Oregano

Smoked paprika

Turmeric

Ground cinnamon

Ground cumin

1 (15-ounce) jar mayonnaise

Mustard (any kind, Dijon recommended)

Tomato paste

Hot sauce (any kind, Tabasco recommended)

Worcestershire sauce

OTHER

32 ounces unsweetened vanilla almond milk

5 to 6 dates

Chia seeds

Flaxseed

Capers

1 small package frozen peas

1 can anchovy fillets

1 (26-ounce) box chicken stock

1 (28-ounce) can crushed tomatoes

1 (14-ounce) can fire-roasted tomatoes

Vanilla extract

Protein powder (see Jen's specs, page 218)

1 can cooking spray (vegetable, coconut, or olive oil)

Prepare

8 *Protein Pancakes (page 210)*

3 servings *Egg Salad (page 228)*

2 *Salmon Bakes (page 276)*

Note: For your *Salmon Bake (page 276),* you will completely set up the dish without actually cooking it today. Prep it in the baking dish, place a lid on it, and refrigerate. The nights these are on your plan, all you need to do is take the lid off, throw them in the oven, and enjoy!

Snack Stash: This week, your daily snack is 1 apple and 1 ounce cashews or walnuts. Pack them with you every day, as they *must* be consumed within each day outside a regular meal. They come in handy when you need to grab some instant nutrition and fight cravings.

MONDAY

BREAKFAST
2 *Protein Pancakes (page 210)*
2 cups strawberries
Watermark: Hit 35 ounces water

LUNCH
Simple Shake #4 (page 223) (increase protein powder to 1^1/$_2$ scoops)
Watermark: Hit 55 ounces water

DINNER
Slow Cooker Shredded Chicken 2.0 (page 280) (over romaine)
Watermark: Hit 75 ounces water (45 minutes before bedtime)

TUESDAY

BREAKFAST
Blueberry Protein Smoothie (page 217)
Watermark: Hit 35 ounces water

LUNCH
Egg Salad (page 228) (^{1}/$_3$ of the recipe, on arugula)
Watermark: Hit 55 ounces water

DINNER
Salmon Bakes (page 276)
Watermark: Hit 75 ounces water (45 minutes before bedtime)

WEDNESDAY

BREAKFAST
2 *Protein Pancakes* (*page 210*)
2 cups strawberries
Watermark: Hit 35 ounces water

LUNCH
Simple Shake #4 (*page 223*) (increase protein powder to
1¹/₂ scoops)
Watermark: Hit 55 ounces water

DINNER
Mama Widerstrom's Grilled Caesar Salad with Skirt Steak
(*page 266*)
Watermark: Hit 75 ounces water (45 minutes before bedtime)

THURSDAY

BREAKFAST
Blueberry Protein Smoothie (*page 217*)
Watermark: Hit 35 ounces water

LUNCH
Egg Salad (*page 228*) (¹/₃ of the recipe, on arugula)
Watermark: Hit 55 ounces water

DINNER
Salmon Bakes (*page 276*)
Watermark: Hit 75 ounces water (45 minutes before bedtime)

FRIDAY

BREAKFAST
2 *Protein Pancakes* (*page 210*)
2 cups strawberries
Watermark: Hit 35 ounces water

LUNCH

Simple Shake #4 (page 223) (increase protein powder to 1½ scoops)

Watermark: Hit 55 ounces water

DINNER

Spicy Stuffed Peppers (page 285)

Watermark: Hit 75 ounces water (45 minutes before bedtime)

SATURDAY

BREAKFAST

Blueberry Protein Smoothie (page 217)

Watermark: Hit 35 ounces water

LUNCH

Egg Salad (page 228) (⅓ of the recipe, on arugula)

Watermark: Hit 55 ounces water

DINNER

One-Pot Cauliflower Rice Paella (page 267)

Watermark: Hit 75 ounces water (45 minutes before bedtime)

SUNDAY

BREAKFAST

2 *Protein Pancakes (page 210)*

2 cups strawberries

Watermark: Hit 35 ounces water

LUNCH

Blueberry Protein Smoothie (page 217)

Watermark: Hit 55 ounces water

DINNER

Shaved Brussels Sprouts Salad (page 238) with *Simple Steak Filet (page 278)*

Watermark: Hit 75 ounces water (45 minutes before bedtime)

Meet Christin

"When I first began working with Jen, I had just had my fourth baby and had essentially spent the past seven years either pregnant or nursing. I was spending all of my time caring for my kids, and it became more difficult to lose the weight after each pregnancy. I had decided it was time to take care of me and gain back my confidence. In the beginning, my goals seemed overwhelming and out of reach, but Jen encouraged me that with consistency, and my body learning to trust me again, that I would see results quickly. The long-term goal I set was to reach my wedding weight (150 pounds) at one year postpregnancy.

"What I like most about my personalized diet is the clear and concise guidelines. It takes out the guesswork. I know what and when to eat to best fuel my body. With some planning and preparation, I can easily stick to it. The way I eat now is more of a lifestyle rather than a crash diet.

"My starting weight was more than 200 pounds. After one month, I was down 8 pounds and 10½ inches all over my body.

"After three months, I had lost 24 pounds and 28 inches all over my body.

"After four months of working with Jen, closely following her nutrition and exercise plan, I got to my pre-baby-number-four weight. I feel strong and healthy again. I've been the girl who has tried every diet out there, and this is the only nutrition plan that I have been able to stick with consistently."

PEP TALK

The road to your success is very simple: be as good to yourself as you are to others, and you will *thrive*. This is easier said than done for someone like you, so please stop overlooking your uncanny ability to get shit done and apply that passion to yourself! Start putting yourself higher on your list, start taking just five minutes in the morning to set yourself up for success, and start celebrating your mini victories each day, because I promise you they will add up to major progress.

Your whole life will bloom: your health, your relationships, and the way you feel about yourself by simply allowing you and others to invest in you. My rock star Everyday Hero, there's a whole layer to you that maybe you've never tapped in to or that has just been buried for a while. . . . Let's shed some light on *that* person and show the world how fit, healthy, and in shape you can be.

CHAPTER 9

THE NEVER-EVER

YOUR PERSONALITY SNAPSHOT

> Cerebral

> Intelligent

> Very clear on your likes and dislikes

> Give up easily

> Efficient/effective when you choose to be

> Your own worst enemy

> Constant justification for eating bad foods

> Fear-based failure thinking keeps you from ever starting a fitness program

> Resistant to facing the reality of poor fitness/health issues

I n all my years of owning a training business and being on TV, I've worked with many Never-Evers. They—and you—are definitely a two-sided coin at times. On one side, you're a good communicator, you're intelligent, and you can expertly apply available knowledge. You are successful in any endeavor when you choose to be. You're future-oriented and a visionary, often appearing to be in a world of your own. You know exactly what to do in order to get in shape and achieve better health, but both goals elude you.

A Never-Ever's greatest obstacle is not other people or what they see and hear, but the six inches between their ears. Their self-talk is filled with disbelief and fear—the fear of thinking they won't ever get there or, if somehow they do, they'll end up relapsing to the start anyway, so why even try? But it's important to point out that Never-Evers are not lazy—in fact, quite the opposite. One of their biggest issues is that they don't want to try something unless they know they'll succeed. They don't like to fail, so it's easier not to try than to try and fail.

So when it comes to this area of your life—dieting—you are a bit of a pessimist. Since you expect to fail on a diet, often it happens. You're less likely to seek solutions for your weight because you believe nothing will work for you anyway.

This sentiment can bring out the procrastinator in you—a tendency that may be harmful to your health. A Canadian study published in the scholarly journal *Personality and Individual Differences* discovered that hard-core procrastinators have more health problems than people who do not procrastinate. Why? It's because procrastinators make a habit out of putting things off; they're less likely to seek medical attention; and they are frequently under a lot of stress. What's more, they don't manage their diet well, and they don't exercise regularly.

When I coach Never-Evers, I have to go about things in a very different way. Instead of developing a course of action for you to follow, I give you a *cause of action*. Securing your commitment to a benefits-based program is the key to you thriving.

That said, let's look at you in the context of your life. Generally, your work life is compartmentalized from your weight issues. At work, you're competent, cooperative, and focused on your career. You bring wisdom and technical skills to the job. Through your knowledge and experiences, you've developed a computer-like sense that lets you quickly sort through information and pull out the crucial aspects.

You like to conceptualize and see things from the perspective of innovation, creativity, and imagination. You're abstract and idealistic but very clear when you make your point. You look at data and read between the lines to find meaning. When dealing with others at work, you think that what's in your brain should be in theirs. If your ideas fall flat, you feel discouraged and resort to sulking. It takes some time, but you're able to pick yourself up.

During your alone time, you often wonder why you're so successful in your career but can't get your body in shape. You've done your research and sincerely want to be healthy—if only wanting it were enough!

You prefer staying at home rather than going out and socializing.

Your home is your haven, and you've created it for personal comfort. You don't have much of a routine at home, but you're good at concentrating on the task at hand.

As a parent, you're warm, accepting, and responsive, but nondemanding. Kids are going to do what they want, right? So why try to lay down the law or exercise too much parental control?

If your spouse or partner is into fitness and exercise, that's a very good thing for you. Support from healthy, successful people in your inner circle has a powerfully positive impact on you. It usually takes some convincing, but once you're sold on the perks of a healthy lifestyle, you begin to match your knowledge base with the use of your emotive passion in a *positive* way, and you're all in.

There are so many things you do well in your life—but nutritional stability is not one of them. You like to eat and drink and not worry about the consequences. Of course, this is probably the reason you're not as thin and fit as maybe you used to be. Your weight has crept on very slowly, until you had that "mirror moment," having no idea how you let things get that far.

When it comes to weight gain, you prefer to stick your head in the sand and ignore the fact that your clothes no longer fit, or that your doctor has told you to shed some pounds. You have developed a habit of dismissing this kind of feedback because for you to acknowledge those facts compels you to act and do something about it. Unfortunately, this attitude is why you keep getting stuck. Burying the thoughts, feelings, and information that are a reflection of your unhappiness and stress separates you even further from the life you really want. You must recognize that there is something wrong in your physical and/or emotional health in order to activate yourself and do something about it. Because you are a Never-Ever, it's you against yourself.

Like most people, you've tried everything from the cabbage soup diet to drinking diet shakes all day, but these regimens never seem to last long. You also possess a skewed perception of effort when it comes to the sacrifices you feel you're making at your meals during these diets. A feeling of "Haven't I given up enough? I at least deserve a little XYZ" is in your headspace every time you eat, and a game of compromises ensues. I'll give you an example. I went out to lunch with one of my Never-Ever clients, and she ordered a fried calamari salad. I looked over and said, "Umm, fried calamari?" With a smirk and a shrug, she replied: "At least it's a salad." She felt that since she had already given up her usual French fries and Diet Coke, why shouldn't she get to keep her calamari?

Often I see Never-Evers holding on to certain foods or meals because you derive emotional satiation from them and experience a corresponding feeling of loss if I ask you to remove them. In a way, at the end of a hard day, or even a hard hour, you feel like food is all you have left.

A NEVER-EVER IN REAL LIFE: ERIN

Erin, age forty-four, was on a path to self-destruction and needed to make some serious course corrections. She was 100 pounds overweight and had given up on dieting and exercise. As a last-ditch effort, she attended a seminar on weight-loss surgery for help.

"I knew that I was overweight, but I always saw it as manageable," she said. "But I had a moment, sitting there with a roomful of obese people. I looked at each of them, judging how fat they were, when I realized we all looked the same—I wasn't just overweight, *I* was officially a fat person. I felt so ashamed because I passed judgment on the others and had ignored my own reality for so long. By the end of the meeting I decided to face that reality and live out my truth."

After realizing that even after the surgery, she'd still have to diet and work out, Erin made up her mind: "I wanted to try it on my own first—at least one more time."

She lost about twenty-five pounds on her own but hired me as her personal trainer and nutrition coach in order to keep going. Her history of trying different diets and going off them filled her with a lot of conflicting directives, so all the misguided information along with her somewhat pessimistic attitude about losing the rest of the weight made it clear she was a Never-Ever. The real downside of this personality is the belief that if they can't do it, they will do nothing. Thus, my priority was to keep her eyes up and feet moving forward, making her connect to every inch of her progress. I also encouraged her to stay educated by subscribing to fitness journals and magazines; reading books, newsletters, and online articles; attending lecture series, workshops, and conferences on obesity and being overweight—the dangers and the solutions—and reading success stories of people who lost weight and kept it off.

Erin lost more weight while also building muscle. She chose activities she liked to do, in addition to our training: dance fitness classes, box and tone training, and Pilates. After three months of working out like this, her entire shape began to noticeably change. She dropped 18 pounds the first month and another 11 the second, and by the third month she had shed a total of 44 pounds. Erin ultimately achieved her goal weight of 155—a weight she was able to maintain for the rest of that year.

It's very hard for Never-Evers like Erin to realize that diet and exercise don't have to be an "I will fail again" proposition. But as she learned, you can be successful with the right tools and the right plan.

THE SUPPORT YOU NEED TO SUCCEED

Out of all the personalities, you require the most support in order to be successful; however, once you take ownership of your journey the sky is the limit.

Until then, and all along your journey, seek out support systems to prop you up. This is critical for you at the beginning to help get you unstuck. Family members, friends, and co-workers can play an important part in helping your efforts to lose weight. Be up-front with what you're taking on and ask that your plans together can start to include healthier lifestyle choices. Suggest an end-of-day workout instead of happy hour, a fun breakfast or even a group hike as your birthday celebration. With your team of people on board, it'll help turn these once difficult decisions into pleasurable executables.

In addition, consider hiring a personal trainer who will have the education to help you achieve fitness goals, safely and efficiently. Invite other friends to go on my plan with you so not only do you have a partner in crime, but you can also start to feel the empowerment that comes from stepping up for somebody else the way they step up for you. That feeling will be synergistic to your efforts going forward. Because you're talking the talk, you're going to *want* to walk the walk. Lean into this!

Within these interactions you'll discover the power of accountability and, more important, of yourself! Allow this mental shift to occur. You're not the only Never-Ever out there; others are on the same path, having the same feelings that you have had, and experiencing the same success that now awaits you.

BEHAVIOR THAT ENCOURAGES WEIGHT GAIN

- Allowing complacency in small tasks, which breeds complacency in bigger ones
- Figuring out meals/workouts in the moment
- Mindless eating/ignoring portions
- Procrastinating
- Talking yourself out of workouts
- Muting how you really feel with food, alcohol, or work

BEHAVIOR THAT ENCOURAGES WEIGHT LOSS

- Honest self-talk
- Developing big-picture goals
- Regular health checkups
- Weighing in daily
- Journaling/daily note-taking
- Scheduling workouts a week out
- Knowing what's in the foods you're eating

THE NEVER-EVER MEAL PLAN

You can be your greatest accomplishment. You simply need to get out of your own way. In the past, your habit has been to manipulate your way through diets and commitments using your own set of jaded reasoning over the one provided with the plan. "I didn't finish all my lunch today so I get to have a bigger dinner." "I feel like I have a cold coming on—I can't work out today because work is really busy right now and I can't afford to get sick." Unfortunately, this only creates disconnected transactions within yourself.

We will change this pattern now. No more starting and stopping. No more quitting. I will disrupt these patterns that have a negative impact on your journey to great health and replace them with ones that promote healthy choices.

Think about a loved one. You know that relationship flourishes when you are connected to their needs. In the same light, you'll create a healthy relationship with your body by anticipating its needs and providing it with nourishment before you get deep into that state of hunger. I will coach you through your isolating patterns, and we will build loyalty toward yourself, and the health changes you make will have staying power and longevity.

Facing the facts fuels you, so I will immerse you in a big-picture plan for each week. Again, my goal for your program is not to give you a course of action but instead to offer you a *cause of action*. Week to week, you'll be given new directives, points of focus, and goals. The weeks themselves will also be unique, oscillating between five and nine days, but still bringing you through a four-week plan.

Your diet is set up in phases—with the first five days designed to jump-start your weight loss. Never-Evers need a sense that they can be successful, so the positive results you'll get right away will motivate you to keep going.

In many ways, you're discovering your identity in a wellness space; therefore, I've allowed room for some personal discovery in your plan. Through this next month, you'll learn about what you lean toward and what makes you thrive. Cooking, with both simplistic and multistep recipes that range from making homemade broths and teas to three-ingredient dinners and prepackaged snacks, will all be included.

Know that I'm not passing any judgment on you for how you ended up here and that you should release any negative judgment that you're carrying for yourself. I'm offering to meet you where you're at *today*. You have a rhythm that is necessary for you, and I'm not looking to disrupt that rhythm but instead honor and support it.

That's a promise.

PHASE 1: THE FIVE-DAY JUMP START

Phase 1 consists of food and beverages that provide anti-inflammatory benefits and promote low acidity. What you put in your body will lower your stress levels and give your insides a much-needed siesta. We start with such a specific menu because it removes the chaos from your digestive system. Artificial "faux foods" such as chips and processed meats are distracting your body from remembering what it was built to do. When you give your body a break from working so hard, it will be ready to receive the changes we are about to make. We are also resetting your body through herbal support and micronutrients with a fiber focus and no dairy—all of which help accelerate weight loss. I will also equip you with two powerful broths as your daily satiating snacks. You should see a significant drop on the scales after five days—an accomplishment that will build your often-flagging confidence and set you on a path toward dieting success that you haven't felt in a long time.

Sipping Snack Options

You will need to make a batch for the next five days. Choose one.

- *Strengthening Bone Broth (page 239):* 5 minutes to prepare/ 10-plus hours to slow-cook

  Bone broth is rich in antioxidants, vitamins, minerals, and gelatin, which are all packed with healing properties and allow your body to utilize complete proteins.

- *Miso Seaweed Detox Broth (page 233)* (this is the vegetarian option): 2 hours to prepare/30 minutes to cook

  Miso has nutrients and minerals that are essential to your body in order for it to function and thrive, such as B vitamins, vitamin K, vitamin E, calcium, iron, and even potassium.

Herbal Support

Have on hand a variety of teas: black, green, chamomile, fennel, ginger, lavender, passionflower, peppermint, and valerian root. I also recommend that you drink a cup of turmeric tea (see page 167) daily as "extra credit." It's popular for its anti-inflammatory and healing properties, dating all the way back to ancient India.

There are several other benefits to enjoying tea on your plan:

Hydration

By drinking these teas throughout the day, you hit 48 ounces of water daily—perfect for hydration and fat burning.

Also, several of these teas—namely chamomile and valerian root—are known to calm anxiety, something that Never-Evers often deal with. Proper hydration, in general, helps your body deal with the effects of stress and anxiety, too.

I advocate tea as a beverage for all my clients because it is a smart, healthy drink that contains no health-destroying additives.

A Calming Activity

Drinking tea can also be a calming activity if you sit down and sip it slowly, almost as if you are meditating. Gaining stillness and relaxation is something anxiety-ridden people need. In other words, no running around with your tea in hand. Take time to enjoy it in a quiet atmosphere. Make this a habit, and it will become very healthy for your spirit.

The Power of Routine

Finally, drinking tea becomes part of a routine, and routines themselves keep you in a better rhythm all day long. To feel dialed into your day is very grounding, so use the routine to stabilize and reset your day.

Hydration Goal

48 ounces (6 cups), minimum, through daily teas

Phase 1 Grocery List

(Many of these ingredients you will use again in future weeks.)

PROTEIN

3 boneless skinless chicken breasts

2 (6-ounce) salmon fillets

PRODUCE

32 ounces berries (blueberries, raspberries, or blackberries)

1 avocado

2 kiwi

5 lemons

DIY Turmeric Tea

Make your own morning brew that is a great substitute for your typical morning cup of coffee. This tea is anti-inflammatory, strengthens digestion, and boosts the immune system.

SERVES 1 TO 2

1 teaspoon ground cinnamon

1 teaspoon fresh ginger

1 teaspoon turmeric

Dash of black pepper (this is necessary to activate the turmeric)

Raw honey or stevia to sweeten

Boil 1 to 2 cups water. Then slowly add the cinnamon, ginger, turmeric, and pepper and simmer for 10 minutes. Strain, if desired, and add honey or stevia. You can also add any nondairy milk such as coconut milk or hemp milk for a creamier drink. Simply mix in ½ cup nondairy milk and blend or whisk with a spoon.

3 limes

1 pear

5 ounces arugula

1 large bundle asparagus

12 ounces broccoli

12 ounces broccolini

1 cup diced carrots

12 ounces cauliflower

1 cup diced celery

1 head garlic

Fresh ginger

10 ounces fresh kale

1 head romaine lettuce

1 small bundle mint

2 cups mushrooms

1 bundle green onions (scallions)

1 yellow onion

10 ounces fresh spinach

2 cups butternut squash

1 cup cherry tomatoes

1 zucchini

DAIRY

None

STARCHES

1 (32-ounce) package short pasta (gluten-free)

1 (32-ounce) package quinoa

NUTS/OILS

6 ounces sliced almonds

1 small package pine nuts

1 medium bottle olive oil

SPICES/CONDIMENTS

Salt

Black pepper

Bay leaves

Ground cinnamon

Thyme, dried

Turmeric

Stevia

Raw honey

Low-sodium soy sauce

OTHER

Dried cranberries

Golden raisins

1 (15-ounce) can white beans

1 small package frozen peas

32 ounces chicken stock

1 small jar pesto

1 (14-ounce) can chopped tomatoes

1 can cooking spray (vegetable, coconut, or olive oil)

TEAS

Black

Chamomile

Fennel

Ginger

Peppermint

Valerian root, lavender, or passionflower

Sipping Snacks: Whether you do the regular or vegetarian option for this phase, add the ingredients of whichever one you choose to this grocery list.

DAY 1

Pack 24 ounces (3 cups) of your sipping snack to be consumed throughout the day.

Upon waking: 16 ounces (2 cups) of digestive support tea with lemon (homemade brew, black, or chamomile)
Note: 16 ounces is just a medium/grande at a coffee shop.

BREAKFAST
Berries and Greens Smoothie (page 216)

LUNCH
Hearty Minestrone Soup (page 230) (1/3 of batch)

AFTERNOON ELIXIR
16 ounces (2 cups) ginger tea

DINNER
Kale Quinoa Chop (page 263)

GOOD NIGHT
16 ounces (2 cups) calming tea (valerian root, lavender, or passionflower tea)

DAY 2

Pack 24 ounces (3 cups) of your sipping snack to be consumed throughout the day.

Upon waking: 16 ounces (2 cups) digestive support tea with lemon (homemade brew, black, or chamomile)
Note: 16 ounces is just a medium/grande at a coffee shop.

BREAKFAST
Pear and Minted Greens Smoothie (page 220)

LUNCH
Roasted Vegetable Salad (page 235)
Note: Make double the recipe so you're set for Day 4!

AFTERNOON ELIXIR
16 ounces (2 cups) fennel tea

DINNER
Ginger-Lime Salmon with Asparagus (page 259)

GOOD NIGHT
  16 ounces (2 cups) calming tea (valerian root, lavender, or
    passionflower tea)

DAY 3

Pack 24 ounces (3 cups) of your sipping snack to be consumed
throughout the day.

Upon waking: 16 ounces (2 cups) digestive support tea with
    lemon (homemade brew, black, or chamomile)
Note: 16 ounces is just a medium/grande at a coffee shop.

BREAKFAST
  Berries and Greens Smoothie (page 216)

LUNCH
  Hearty Minestrone Soup (page 230) (1/3 of batch)

AFTERNOON ELIXIR
  16 ounces (2 cups) peppermint tea

DINNER
  Zucchini Pesto Pasta Sauté (page 293) (with chicken)

GOOD NIGHT
  16 ounces (2 cups) calming tea (valerian root, lavender, or
    passionflower tea)

DAY 4

Pack 24 ounces (3 cups) of your sipping snack to be consumed
throughout the day.

Upon waking: 16 ounces (2 cups) digestive support tea with
    lemon (homemade brew, black or chamomile)
Note: 16 ounces is just a medium/grande at a coffee shop.

BREAKFAST
  Pear and Minted Greens Smoothie (page 220)

LUNCH
Roasted Vegetable Salad (page 235) (use second batch from Day 2)

AFTERNOON ELIXIR
16 ounces (2 cups) fennel tea

DINNER
Pan-Seared Salmon with Garlicky Kale (page 272)

GOOD NIGHT
16 ounces (2 cups) calming tea (valerian root, lavender, or
passionflower tea)

DAY 5

Pack 24 ounces (3 cups) of your sipping snack to be consumed
throughout the day.

Upon waking: 16 ounces (2 cups) digestive support tea with
lemon (homemade brew, black, or chamomile)
Note: 16 ounces is just a medium/grande at a coffee shop.

BREAKFAST
Berries and Greens Smoothie (page 216)

LUNCH
Hearty Minestrone Soup (page 230) (last 1/3 of batch)

AFTERNOON ELIXIR
16 ounces (2 cups) ginger tea

DINNER
Spring Greens Super Salad (page 286)

GOOD NIGHT
16 ounces (2 cups) calming tea (valerian root, lavender, or
passionflower tea)

PHASE 2: THE NINE-DAY REBOOT AND ENERGIZE

During Phase 2, I've added in several more nourishing foods, greater nutritional variety, and healthy carbs. Variety, not restriction, means a healthier diet. It also means a diet with a greater success rate. In 2014, Harvard researchers found that greater healthful food variety may protect against weight gain, plus it helped men and women lose excess belly fat.

You'll also be "cycling" your carbs during this phase. This means that on certain days, you'll eat carbs at every meal; on other days, you'll follow a lower-carb menu. Carbohydrate cycling is an excellent way to keep your body in a fat-burning, muscle-building mode. If you eat carbs on a continual basis, your body gets accustomed to breaking them down quickly, because carbs are your body's first choice when it comes to fuel. The energy from carbs is important for getting through intense workouts and ultimately building lean muscle. But when you periodically decrease carb intake, your body relies on burning fat for fuel instead. So with carb cycling, you get the best of both worlds: more curvy muscle and less jiggly fat.

Carb cycling has been verified scientifically, too. In a four-month study, British researchers found that people who cycled their carbs lost an average of nine pounds of fat compared with five pounds lost by those following a standard calorie-controlled diet.

Hydration Goal
64 ounces water daily

Phase 2 Grocery List
(Many of these ingredients may be left over from Phase 1. Recheck your stash before buying more.)

PROTEIN

14 large eggs

1 boneless skinless chicken breast

2 (5-ounce) cans chicken (water packed; organic is best)

1 (6-ounce) turkey patty

14 ounces sliced turkey deli meat

4 ounces sliced ham

1 (6-ounce) beef patty

12 ounces skirt steak

1 pound halibut fillets

2 (6-ounce) salmon fillets

1 (6-ounce) tuna steak fillet

PRODUCE

1 apple

1 avocado

1 banana

18 ounces blueberries

6 ounces raspberries

16 ounces strawberries

1 pear

2 lemons

5 ounces arugula

2 cups broccoli

12 cups (32 ounces) Brussels sprouts

2 cups diced carrots

2 cups cauliflower

1 small bunch celery

1 cucumber

6 to 8 Persian cucumbers

1 head romaine lettuce

1 red onion

1 yellow onion

2 cups snap peas

5 ounces fresh spinach

1/2 pint cherry tomatoes

3 to 4 tomatoes (such as Roma or heirloom)

DAIRY

2 cups 2% Greek yogurt

STARCHES

1 medium container (18 ounces) old-fashioned oats (see Jen's specs, page 85)

1 loaf sprouted bread

14 ounces black rice

1 (32-ounce) package brown rice

32 ounces quinoa

1 large sweet potato

NUTS/OILS

6 ounces sliced almonds

16 ounces cashews

16 ounces walnuts

1 medium bottle olive oil

SPICES/CONDIMENTS

Salt

Black pepper

Chili powder

Garlic powder

Onion powder

Oregano, dried

Parsley, dried

Thyme, dried

Paprika

Barbecue sauce

Red wine vinegar

Soy sauce (regular or low-sodium)

Tabasco sauce

Ketchup (optional)
Mustard
Mayonnaise
Butter
Tomato paste
Honey

OTHER

Unsweetened vanilla almond
    milk (or 2% milk)
Golden raisins
5 dates
Chia seeds
Pomegranate seeds
Sesame seeds
Capers
Pickles (optional)
1 (15-ounce) can chickpeas
Clam juice
Dry white wine
Protein powder (see Jen's
    specs, page 218)
1 can cooking spray (vegetable,
    coconut, or olive oil)

DAY 1

(Eat carbs at every meal—we want to hit 150 to 200 grams starch carbs—but little to no fat today.)

Upon waking: 8 ounces (1 cup) water

BREAKFAST

1½ cups cooked oatmeal with 1 cup blueberries
16 ounces (2 cups) water

LUNCH

Grilled Tuna with Brown Rice and Veggies (page 229)
16 ounces (2 cups) water

AFTERNOON SNACK

1 pear
16 ounces (2 cups) water

DINNER

Protein-Style Turkey Burger with Cubed Sweet Potatoes (page 274)
8 ounces (1 cup) water

DAY 2

Upon waking: 8 ounces (1 cup) water

BREAKFAST
Ham and Avocado Frittata *(page 205)*
16 ounces (2 cups) water

LUNCH
Chicken Salad Romaine Wraps (page 224)
16 ounces (2 cups) water

AFTERNOON SNACK
Simple Shake #1 (page 222)
16 ounces (2 cups) water

DINNER
Fish Stew (page 256)
8 ounces (1 cup) water

DAY 3

Repeat Day 2.

DAY 4

(Eat carbs at every meal—we want to hit 150 to 200 grams starch carbs—but little to no fat today.)

Upon waking: 8 ounces (1 cup) water

BREAKFAST
$1\frac{1}{2}$ cups cooked oatmeal with 1 cup blueberries
16 ounces (2 cups) water

LUNCH
Turkey sandwich made with 5 ounces deli turkey, any leafy lettuce, tomato, and mustard on 2 slices sprouted bread. (No fat-based toppings like cheese, mayonnaise, or avocado.)
16 ounces (2 cups) water

AFTERNOON SNACK
1 apple
16 ounces (2 cups) water

DINNER
Burger Patty with Veggie Quinoa Salad (page 251)
8 ounces (1 cup) water

DAY 5

Upon waking: 8 ounces (1 cup) water

BREAKFAST
Protein Smoothie with Red Berries (page 222)
16 ounces (2 cups) water

LUNCH
Shaved Brussels Sprouts Salad (page 238)
16 ounces (2 cups) water

AFTERNOON SNACK
2 hard-boiled eggs
16 ounces (2 cups) water

DINNER
Baked Sesame Salmon with Roasted Veggies (page 243)
8 ounces (1 cup) water

DAY 6

Repeat Day 5.

DAY 7

(Eat carbs at every meal—we want to hit 150 to 200 grams starch carbs—but NO fat today.)

Upon waking: 8 ounces (1 cup) water

BREAKFAST
1½ cups cooked oatmeal with 1 cup blueberries
16 ounces (2 cups) water

LUNCH
*Protein-Style Turkey Burger with Cubed Sweet Potatoes
(page 274)*
16 ounces (2 cups) water

AFTERNOON SNACK
1 banana
16 ounces (2 cups) water

DINNER
BBQ Baked Chicken (page 245)
8 ounces (1 cup) water

DAY 8

Upon waking: 8 ounces (1 cup) water

BREAKFAST
1 cup 2% Greek yogurt with ¼ cup walnuts or sliced almonds,
drizzled with honey
16 ounces (2 cups) water

LUNCH
Egg Salad (page 228) (on arugula)
16 ounces (2 cups) water

AFTERNOON SNACK
4 ounces sliced turkey deli meat roll-ups
16 ounces (2 cups) water

DINNER
Skirt Steak and Roasted Brussels Sprouts (page 278)
8 ounces (1 cup) water

DAY 9

Repeat Day 8.

PHASE 3: THE FIVE-DAY LEAN-DOWN

The mission of this phase is to create an even more ingrained rhythm that your body can trust and open up to. When you establish this trust, your body will shed even more weight because, believe it or not, it doesn't want to be fat, either! Often, our bodies get stuck in fight-or-flight mode because of our inconsistent decisions. This phase will officially pull you out of that mode. We'll accomplish this through specific nutritional timing of a higher volume of nutrient-dense greens, increased fats, and minimal dairy.

You will eat every 2½ hours, including highly digestible proteins—a pattern that will fire up your metabolism so that your body is burning its fat tank at peak efficiency to create a leaner you.

Hydration Goal:

72 ounces (9 cups) water daily by drinking 12 ounces (1½ cups) water before every meal.

Phase 3 Grocery List

(Many of these ingredients may be left over from Phases 1 and 2. Re-check your stash before buying more.)

PROTEIN

10 large eggs

2 boneless skinless chicken breasts

12 ounces protein for *DIY Stir-Fry (page 254)*

(chicken, shrimp, steak, or vegetarian)

1 (6-ounce) beef patty

2 (5-ounce) cans tuna (water packed)

PRODUCE

4 apples

1 avocado

12 ounces blueberries

16 ounces strawberries

4 lemons

1 small package basil

1 cup broccoli

12 ounces green beans

1 bunch celery

1 small bundle chives

Collard greens, big leaves

3 cucumbers

6 cups edamame (fresh or frozen)

1 head garlic

10 ounces fresh kale

1 head romaine lettuce

1 cup mushrooms

1 Vidalia onion

5 ounces fresh spinach

2 tomatoes

6 cups Asian veggies for *DIY Stir-Fry* (*page 254*)

DAIRY

2 cups 2% Greek yogurt

1 package sliced cheese (any kind)

1 block Parmesan cheese, to be grated

STARCHES

1 medium container (18 ounces) old-fashioned oats (see Jen's specs, page 85)

1 box granola (see Jen's specs, page 85)

NUTS/OILS

16 ounces almonds

16 ounces pecans

1 small package macadamia nuts

1 small package pine nuts

1 medium jar peanut or almond butter

1 medium bottle olive oil

SPICES/CONDIMENTS

Salt

Black pepper

Cayenne pepper

Red pepper flakes

Parsley, dried

Rosemary, fresh or dried

Apple cider vinegar

White wine vinegar

Hot sauce (any kind)

Soy sauce (regular or low-sodium)

Mustard (any kind)

Honey or agave

OTHER

32 ounces unsweetened vanilla almond milk (or 2% milk)

1 small package chia seeds

1 (250-gram) package algae powder (spirulina/chlorella) (order from www.watershed.net)

1 container (2 pounds) protein powder (whey, pea, hemp, and nondairy are all acceptable)

1 can cooking spray (vegetable, coconut, or olive oil)

DAY 1

STARTER
Protein Oats 2.0 (page 209)

2¹/₂ HOURS LATER
2 hard-boiled eggs

2¹/₂ HOURS LATER
Greens Juice (page 220)

2¹/₂ HOURS LATER
1 tablespoon peanut or almond butter with 2 to 3 celery stalks

2¹/₂ HOURS LATER
Grilled Herbed Chicken with Spicy String Beans (page 260)

2¹/₂ HOURS LATER
2 cups edamame (lightly salted)

DAY 2

STARTER
Greek Yogurt and Fruit (page 202)

2¹/₂ HOURS LATER
Simple Shake #2 (page 222)

2¹/₂ HOURS LATER
Tuna Salad Wraps (page 240) (in collard greens)

2¹/₂ HOURS LATER
Handful of almonds

2¹/₂ HOURS LATER
DIY Stir-Fry (page 254)

2¹/₂ HOURS LATER
Veggie Scramble (page 212)

DAY 3

STARTER
Protein Oats 2.0 (page 209)

2¹/₂ HOURS LATER
2 hard-boiled eggs

2¹/₂ HOURS LATER
Greens Juice (page 220)

2¹/₂ HOURS LATER
1 tablespoon peanut or almond butter with 2 to 3 celery stalks

2¹/₂ HOURS LATER
Burger Bowl (page 250)

2¹/₂ HOURS LATER
2 cups edamame (lightly salted)

DAY 4

STARTER
Greek Yogurt and Fruit (page 202)

2¹/₂ HOURS LATER
Simple Shake #2 (page 222)

2¹/₂ HOURS LATER
Tuna Salad Wraps (page 240) (in collard greens)

2¹/₂ HOURS LATER
Handful of almonds

2¹/₂ HOURS LATER
DIY Stir-Fry (page 254)

2¹/₂ HOURS LATER
Veggie Scramble (page 212)

DAY 5

STARTER
Protein Oats 2.0 (page 209)

2¹/₂ HOURS LATER
2 hard-boiled eggs

2¹/₂ HOURS LATER
Greens Juice (page 220)

2¹/₂ HOURS LATER
1 tablespoon peanut or almond butter with 2 to 3 celery stalks

2¹/₂ HOURS LATER
Cranberry Nut Kale Salad (page 253) (with 6 ounces grilled chicken)

2¹/₂ HOURS LATER
2 cups edamame (lightly salted)

PHASE 4: FINAL NINE—STRONG AND STEADY

In this final phase, I give you a new nutritional blueprint, featuring a livable life rhythm that is replicable and, dare I say, *enjoyable!* Stamina and consistency are the focus in putting mental/emotional energy toward your nutritional execution. You'll notice the continued inclusion of one-ingredient foods that your body identifies quickly and easily digests to keep your metabolism firing.

We'll also be going green (and red, orange, white, and purple) because I'm adding even more variety and I'll ask that you include a few vegetarian meals this week. I find that many of my clients aren't as skilled in preparing vegetable dishes as they are with protein. This challenge (to some) encourages culinary creativity. When I started this type of regimen, I stuck to the basics: broccoli, asparagus, and Brussels sprouts. Now I've expanded my repertoire to include the preparation of pumpkin, chard, eggplant, and parsnip, among other veggies. By investing some time in a "veg-education," you'll begin to appreciate veggies even more, plus develop some killer kitchen skills. Going all-veggie gives your body a deserved reprieve from saturated fat and cholesterol and is a great way to flood your system with fiber and micronutrients. But for those of you who prefer not to go vegetarian, I give you options at meals.

This is the home stretch; now make me proud!

Hydration Goal

72 to 80 ounces (9 to 10 cups) daily through teas and water checkpoints.

Phase 4 Grocery List

(Many of these ingredients may be left over from Phases 1, 2, and 3. Recheck your stash before buying more.)

PROTEIN

12 large eggs

8 to 9 boneless skinless chicken breasts

12 ounces 93% lean ground turkey

12 ounces ground bison

12 ounces skirt steak

12 ounces deli meat (Jen's specs: prioritize organic, nitrate-free brands)

5 ounces salmon fillet

6 ounces sushi-grade tuna

6 ounces shrimp or scallops

6 ounces protein of your choice for *DIY Stir-Fry* (*page 254*)

PRODUCE

2 apples

2 avocados

1 small banana

1 beet

16 ounces fresh berries

3 lemons

1 large bundle asparagus

1 small package basil

6 ounces bean sprouts

1 green bell pepper

1 cup broccoli

1 cup broccolini

1 small package shaved Brussels sprouts

10 ounces shredded carrots

1 small cucumber

6 to 8 Persian cucumbers

16 ounces edamame (fresh or frozen)

1 head garlic

2 cups fresh kale

1 head butter lettuce

3 heads romaine lettuce

5 ounces mixed greens

1 small package mushrooms

1 small bundle green onions (scallions)

1 Vidalia onion

5 ounces spinach

1 spaghetti squash

1 pint cherry tomatoes

1 tomato (such as Roma or heirloom)

3 cups assorted Asian veggies for *DIY Stir-Fry* (*page 254*)

2 zucchini

DAIRY

2 cups 2% Greek yogurt

1 package sliced cheese (any)

16 ounces cottage cheese

1 block Parmesan cheese, to be grated

STARCHES

1 medium container (18 ounces) old-fashioned oats (see Jen's specs, page 85)

1 loaf sprouted bread

32 ounces brown rice

10 ounces almond or buckwheat flour (optional)

6-inch whole-wheat tortillas

NUTS/OILS

6 ounces sliced almonds

Single-serving packaged nuts (any kind; Trader Joe's has almonds and cashews)

1 medium bottle olive oil

SPICES/CONDIMENTS

Salt

Black pepper

Lemon pepper

Garlic powder

Onion powder

Parsley, dried

Sage leaves

Paprika

Ground cinnamon

Balsamic vinegar

Rice wine vinegar

Hot sauce (Tabasco recommended)

Soy sauce (regular or low-sodium)

Worcestershire sauce

Dijon mustard (Grey Poupon recommended)

Butter

Honey or agave

Vanilla extract

OTHER

32 ounces unsweetened
   vanilla almond milk

30 ounces coconut water

1 small package sesame seeds

1 small package shelled
   sunflower seeds

1 can anchovy fillets

11 ounces hummus

Dill pickles (optional)

1 (13-ounce) jar low-sugar or
   low-carb marinara sauce

1 jar pesto

1 container (2 pounds)
   protein powder (whey,
   pea, hemp, and nondairy
   all acceptable) (see Jen's
   specs, page 218)

1 can cooking spray
   (vegetable, coconut, or
   olive oil)

TEAS

Black, ginger, and/or
   chamomile

Peppermint

Valerian root, fennel, and/or
   passionflower

DAYS 1 AND 2

Upon waking: 12 ounces (1½ cups) water

BREAKFAST

1 slice sprouted bread, with ½ tablespoon butter

2 hard-boiled eggs

1 apple

A.M. TEA

20 ounces (2½ cups) black, ginger, or chamomile tea

LUNCH

Chicken Wrap #1 (page 225)

12 ounces (1½ cups) water

OR

Chicken Wrap #2 (page 226) (chicken optional, but then add more
   greens, a vegetable protein, and hummus)

12 ounces (1½ cups) water

AFTERNOON SNACK

1 snack-size package of nuts

DINNER
Bison Meatballs and Roasted Spaghetti Squash (page 248)
12 ounces (1¹/₂ cups) water

P.M. TEA
20 ounces (2¹/₂ cups) valerian root, fennel, or passionflower tea

DAY 3 (NO STARCH CARBS)

Upon waking: 12 ounces (1¹/₂ cups) water

BREAKFAST
1 cup 2% Greek yogurt with ¹/₄ cup sliced almonds, drizzled with honey or agave

A.M. TEA
20 ounces (2¹/₂ cups) black or peppermint tea

LUNCH
Seared Ahi Tuna Salad (page 237)
12 ounces (1¹/₂ cups) water

AFTERNOON SNACK
2 cups edamame

DINNER
One-Pot Chicken (page 269) (with broiled asparagus)
12 ounces (1¹/₂ cups) water

P.M. TEA
20 ounces (2¹/₂ cups) valerian root or lavender tea

DAYS 4 AND 5

Upon waking: 12 ounces (1¹/₂ cups) water

BREAKFAST
1 cup cooked oatmeal
¹/₂ cup fresh berries
Protein shake of 1 cup water and 1 scoop protein powder

20 ounces (2 1/2 cups) black, ginger, or chamomile tea

LUNCH
Open-Faced Deli Sammy (page 233)
12 ounces (1 1/2 cups) water

AFTERNOON SNACK
1 snack-size package of nuts

DINNER
*Mama Widerstrom's Grilled Caesar Salad with Skirt Steak
(page 266) (6 ounces)*
12 ounces (1 1/2 cups) water

P.M. TEA
20 ounces (2 1/2 cups) valerian root, fennel, or passionflower tea

DAY 6 (NO STARCH CARBS)

Upon waking: 12 ounces (1 1/2 cups) water

BREAKFAST
Green Frittata (page 203)

A.M. TEA
20 ounces (2 1/2 cups) black or peppermint tea

LUNCH
Kale and Romaine Chop (page 231) (add 1 to 2 hard-boiled eggs or
4 ounces chicken if you prefer not to go vegetarian)
12 ounces (1 1/2 cups) water

AFTERNOON SNACK
1/2 avocado with lemon and salt

DINNER
Zucchini Pesto Pasta Sauté (page 293) (add shrimp, scallops, or
chicken, optional)
12 ounces (1 1/2 cups) water

20 ounces (2¹/₂ cups) valerian root or lavender tea

DAYS 7 AND 8

Upon waking: 12 ounces (1¹/₂ cups) water

BREAKFAST
2 *Protein Pancakes (page 210)*

A.M. TEA
20 ounces (2¹/₂ cups) black, ginger, or chamomile tea

LUNCH
Chicken and Rice Bowl: 6 ounces cooked chicken served over assorted grilled veggies and 1 cup brown rice (optional: season with soy, garlic, chili oil, or hot sauce)

12 ounces (1¹/₂ cups) water

OR

Vegetarian Rice Bowl: unlimited bok choy, broccoli, carrots, artichokes, water chestnuts, and/or any other vegetables over 1 cup brown rice (optional: season with soy, garlic, chili oil, or hot sauce)

12 ounces (1¹/₂ cups) water

AFTERNOON SNACK
1 snack-size package of nuts

DINNER
Burger Bowl (page 250) (turkey, beef, or vegetarian protein)
12 ounces (1¹/₂ cups) water

P.M. TEA
20 ounces (2¹/₂ cups) valerian root, fennel, or passionflower tea

DAY 9 (NO STARCH CARBS)

Upon waking: 12 ounces (1¹/₂ cups) water

BREAKFAST
Protein-Kale Smoothie (page 221)

A.M. TEA
   20 ounces (2¹/₂ cups) black or peppermint tea

LUNCH
   Salmon Burgers on Butter Lettuce (page 236)
   12 ounces (1¹/₂ cups) water

AFTERNOON SNACK
   ¹/₂ cup cottage cheese

DINNER
   DIY Stir-Fry (page 254)
   12 ounces (1¹/₂ cups) water

P.M. TEA
   20 ounces (2¹/₂ cups) valerian root or lavender tea

Meet Jeanette

"I was beyond excited to start my training with Jen. I knew it would be challenging, but I was determined and made a commitment to myself to get healthy, even though I hadn't been very successful in the past.

"Well, with the Never-Ever meal plan, I was finally successful. The diet recommendations were easy, and the food was delicious. I learned how to stay away from anything processed and go with natural foods.

"The hardest part about the workouts was cardio for me; however, with each session, I saw myself get a little bit stronger, and I could do a little bit more each time. As I got better, the workouts got harder; Jen always kept me on my toes and switched my workouts every time.

"I dropped weight quickly on this plan, and my body didn't fight it at all. I believe that the rapid loss at the start motivated me to keep going. When we began, I weighed 138 pounds and after the program, I was down to 125!

"Jen changed my life. I am forever grateful!"

PEP TALK

I would say this to your face one million times over if I could: "YOU GOT THIS!" And then I would hug you for an uncomfortably long period of time until you hugged me back just as hard. For now, though, my Never-Ever, you will have to settle for my air hug instead, but please feel the belief that I have in you through it. Look at the big picture and let that be your fuel in your day-to-day life.

By taking a macro approach to your diet plan, you will find that the emotion that once kept you feeling stuck will now bring out the momentum, strength, and passion in you. You will feel invigorated in the very first week of this program, and each week afterward will challenge and inspire you to take it head-on.

Even though I want you looking at the big picture, do not look too far down the road. I want you focusing on the week, the day, or even just the meal right in front of you. Take on one thing at a time, master it, and move forward. This will be your mantra that leads you to your goal weight and happiest heart.

CHAPTER 10

RECIPES FOR WEIGHT LOSS AND BEYOND

EGGS, MUFFINS, AND MORE 197

EVERYDAY ENTRÉES   242

T his chapter includes more than 120 recipes to help you on your weight-loss journey and beyond. After your initial four weeks on the plan—or once you've reached your weight-loss goal—you can feel free to use all of the recipes here. Cooking your own meals is one of the best ways to maintain a healthy lifestyle, and as you will see with the recipes here, cooking doesn't have to be a chore; with a few simple guidelines and basic ingredients you can create tons of meals you'll love.

Using fresh ingredients is one of the best secrets to whipping up delicious meals. Always have fresh fruits and veggies on hand, lean meats and seafood in your fridge, and whole grains in your pantry. Follow the nutritional guidelines from Chapter 3 and living healthier will be easier than you ever thought possible.

Enhancing the flavors of your foods is key to not only enjoying them but sustaining these healthy meal combinations in your diet plan. The following is what I call your "Yum-Yum List," because these are all Jen-approved items that will make each bite more delicious than the last *without* compromising your progress on your waistline. (Rebels, these lists will be familiar to you, as they are a fully approved part of your individualized plan.)

BASIC SEASONINGS

Salt	Garlic powder
Black pepper	Onion powder
Lemon pepper	Ground cumin
Red pepper flakes	Paprika (regular or smoked)
Chili powder	Turmeric

When it comes to bread and tortillas, all things are not equal; the following are my simple guidelines.

There's bread in the freezer section of your grocery store that's nutritionally superior to any bread you'll find: sprouted bread. It is baked with whole grains whose seeds have sprouted but not fully germinated; also, the grain is not pulverized into flour, leading to several health benefits. Sprouted breads are higher in vitamin C, folate, minerals like iron, and fiber. The sprouting process also yields a reduction in carbs, along with an increase in protein. Finally, these breads have lower levels of gluten and up to three times the amount of soluble fiber found in nonsprouted grains, making these breads a healthier alternative to white-flour or whole-grain-flour breads.

HERBS—DRIED AND/OR FRESH

Basil

Chives

Cilantro

Dill

Garlic

Oregano

Parsley

Rosemary

Sage

Thyme

CONDIMENTS

Ketchup—limited

Mustard (all kinds)

Mayonnaise—limited

Hummus

Barbecue sauce—limited

Hot sauce (all kinds)

MISCELLANEOUS

Pickles

Lemon

Lime

Apple cider vinegar

Balsamic vinegar

Coconut oil

Olive oil

Soy sauce

Chia seeds

Hemp seeds

Agave

Honey

Cooking spray (vegetable, olive, or coconut oil)

You'll find all my favorite recipes here and tons more healthy eating tips, too. Be sure to flip through the entire section to discover everything you need to begin your healthy eating journey. Enjoy!

EGGS, MUFFINS, AND MORE

BANANA WALNUT MUFFINS

MAKES 6 MUFFINS

Olive oil or coconut oil cooking spray

2 large bananas

1 large egg, beaten

1/2 cup spelt flour (available at Whole Foods)

1/2 teaspoon vanilla extract

1/2 tablespoon honey

1/2 teaspoon ground cinnamon

1/2 teaspoon baking soda

1/2 teaspoon salt

1/4 cup finely chopped raw walnuts

Preheat the oven to 375°F. Lightly spray 6 muffin cups with the cooking spray.

In a medium bowl, mash the bananas, then add the beaten egg and combine.

In a separate bowl, combine the flour, vanilla, honey, cinnamon, baking soda, and salt.

Slowly add the flour mixture to the banana mixture and mix, then fold in the walnuts.

Divide the batter evenly among the 6 prepared muffin cups (about two thirds full).

Bake for 25 to 30 minutes, until golden brown or until a wooden toothpick inserted in the center of a muffin comes out clean. Remove from the oven and allow to cool in the pan for 10 minutes before serving.

NOTE
You can store these muffins at room temperature for up to 3 days, or put a portion of these in your refrigerator for later in the week.

BLACK BEAN EGG SCRAMBLE

SERVES 1

Vegetable oil cooking spray
2 large eggs, beaten
2 large egg whites, beaten
3/4 cup black beans
1/2 avocado, pitted, peeled, and chopped
2 to 4 tablespoons pico de gallo

Spray a medium saucepan with the cooking spray. Add the eggs, egg whites, black beans, and avocado and scramble over medium heat. Cook until the eggs are well set. Serve with pico de gallo.

CHEESE AND SPINACH OMELET

SERVES 1

2 large eggs
1 large egg white
Vegetable oil cooking spray
Handful of chopped fresh spinach
1 ounce cheese

In a small bowl, whisk together the eggs and egg white. Spray a small skillet with the cooking spray, then add the egg mixture and spinach.

Cook over medium heat until the eggs are just firm and the spinach is tender. Add the cheese and allow it to melt. Flip one half of the mixture over to form the omelet. Serve.

CRUNCHY OATS

SERVES 1

1 cup cooked oatmeal
1/4 cup granola (see Jen's specs, page 85)
1/2 cup blueberries
14 walnut halves

Combine all the ingredients in a small bowl. Mix well and serve.

EGG AND POTATO SCRAMBLE

SERVES 1

3/4 cup diced regular or sweet potatoes
Salt and pepper, to taste
2 large eggs, beaten
1 large egg white, beaten
1/4 cup shredded Cheddar or mozzarella cheese
Large handful of fresh spinach
Hot sauce (optional)

In a lightly oil-sprayed pan over medium heat, brown the diced potatoes. Season with salt and pepper. Add the eggs and egg white and let them cook through. Stir in the cheese and spinach, and cook until the cheese has melted and the spinach is tender. Season with hot sauce (if using) and serve.

EGG BAKES

SERVES 6

Vegetable oil cooking spray

FOR THE SAUSAGE

1 tablespoon olive oil

1/4 medium yellow onion, finely chopped

1 garlic clove, minced

1/4 pound 93% lean ground turkey

1 teaspoon dried oregano

1 teaspoon fennel seeds

1 teaspoon dried basil

1 teaspoon dried parsley

1/2 teaspoon salt

1/2 teaspoon pepper

FOR THE BAKES

1 cup finely chopped broccoli

1/2 cup shredded Cheddar cheese

2 tablespoons sun-dried tomatoes (soaked in oil), finely chopped

1 teaspoon dried basil

1/4 teaspoon dried oregano

1/2 teaspoon onion powder

1/2 teaspoon sea salt

4 large eggs

1 1/2 teaspoons chopped chives

Preheat the oven to 350°F. Lightly spray 6 muffin cups with cooking spray.

To make the sausage: In a skillet over medium heat, heat the olive oil and cook the onion and garlic for 5 minutes, or until the onion has browned and softened. Remove from the skillet, set aside, and let cool. In a medium bowl, combine the turkey, oregano, fennel, basil, parsley, salt, pepper, and the onion mixture. Mix with your hands until thoroughly blended.

Form patties of the desired width and thickness (3 inches wide by 1/2 to 3/4 inch thick works well) by hand. Cook in a skillet over medium heat, flipping midway, until the meat is no longer pink.

Set the patties aside to cool, then chop and crumble them into bite-size pieces. This creates the "sausage."

To make the bakes: In a large bowl, combine the sausage, broccoli, cheese, tomatoes, basil, oregano, onion powder, and salt.

In a medium bowl, whisk the eggs. Pour the eggs into the broccoli mixture and mix thoroughly. Divide the mixture evenly among the 6 prepared muffin cups and top with the chives.

Bake for 30 minutes or until a wooden toothpick inserted in the center of an egg bake comes out clean. Remove from the oven and allow to cool in the pan for 10 minutes before serving. Store in the refrigerator.

GARDEN OMELET

SERVES 1

2 large eggs
2 large egg whites
Vegetable oil cooking spray
1/2 avocado, pitted, peeled, and chopped
1 cup chopped broccoli
Handful of chopped fresh spinach
1 slice sprouted bread (Ezekiel) or wheat bread,
     toasted

In a small bowl, whisk together the eggs and egg whites. Spray a small skillet with the cooking spray and add the egg mixture, avocado, broccoli, and spinach. Cook over medium heat until the eggs are just firm and the veggies are tender. Flip one half of the mixture over to form the omelet. Serve over the toast.

GGPS (GLUTEN-FREE GREEN PANCAKES)

SERVES 1

1 cup protein powder
1/2 cup brown rice flour
2 teaspoons baking powder
2 cups fresh spinach
1 banana
1 large egg, beaten
1 cup whole milk
Vegetable oil cooking spray

Place all the ingredients except the cooking spray in a blender and pulse until well incorporated. Pour 4 to 5 tablespoons of batter into a lightly oil-sprayed pan or griddle over medium-low heat, so the pancakes don't burn but are still able to cook. Cook for 3 to 4 minutes; when the pancakes begin to bubble, gently flip them over and cook for another 2 to 3 minutes. Serve.

> **JEN JUJU: Brown Rice Flour Power**
> *I've started using brown rice flour for baking, and I love the fluffy texture it lends to baked goods. But more than that, I love the fact that brown rice has fewer calories than wheat flour, has more amino acids, and is gluten-free (which makes it an excellent substitute for wheat when going gluten-free in your diet). You can substitute brown rice flour, cup for cup, for other flours, so the next time you get the urge to bake, go with this nutritious option.*

GREEK YOGURT AND FRUIT

SERVES 1

1 cup 2% Greek yogurt
1 tablespoon chia seeds

1 cup sliced strawberries

Honey or agave, for garnish (optional)

Combine the yogurt, chia seeds, and strawberries in a small bowl. Mix together. Garnish with a thin ribbon of honey or agave (if using) and serve.

JEN JUJU: Go Greek

Greek yogurt is definitely my number one go-to dairy product, and as you can see, I use it in quite a few recipes—and not just for its creamy taste and consistency,

It is filled with vitamins and minerals that your body needs—like vitamin B6, vitamin B12, zinc, potassium, and calcium. The probiotic content of Greek yogurt also helps improve your digestion and is beneficial if you've got tummy troubles.

Greek yogurt is also high in protein—nearly twice the protein of regular yogurt. Another bonus: A 2013 study in Appetite found that an afternoon snack of Greek yogurt can make you feel full and satiated.

GREEN FRITTATA

SERVES 1

2 large eggs

1 large egg white

1/4 teaspoon salt

1/4 teaspoon pepper

1 tablespoon olive oil

1 small shallot, diced

1 small zucchini, diced

1/2 green bell pepper, chopped

Large handful of chopped fresh spinach

1/2 avocado, pitted, peeled, and diced

Preheat the oven to 325°F.

In a small bowl, beat the eggs and egg white with the salt and pepper until light and fluffy, then set them aside.

Heat the olive oil in a small oven-safe pan over medium heat. Add the shallot, zucchini, and bell pepper and cook for 6 to 8 minutes, until soft. Add the spinach and cook for about 1 minute, until it just begins to wilt.

Remove from the heat, pour the egg mixture into the pan, and stir until the eggs are distributed evenly. Put the pan in the oven and cook for 10 to 12 minutes, or until the center is set. Remove from the oven and top with diced avocado. Serve.

GREEN OMELET

SERVES 1

2 large eggs
1 large egg white
Vegetable oil cooking spray
1/2 green bell pepper, chopped
Handful of chopped fresh spinach
1/2 avocado, pitted, peeled, and diced
1/4 cup shredded cheese

In a small bowl, whisk together eggs and egg white. Spray a small skillet with the cooking spray and add the egg mixture, vegetables, and avocado. Cook over medium heat until the eggs are just firm and veggies are tender. Add the cheese and allow it to melt. Flip one half of the mixture over to form the omelet. Serve.

HAM AND AVOCADO FRITTATA

SERVES 1

1 teaspoon olive oil
2 ounces ham, sliced
1/4 cup cherry tomatoes
2 eggs, beaten
Handful of fresh spinach
1/2 avocado, pitted, peeled, and diced
Pinch of salt
Pinch of pepper

Heat the olive oil in a medium saucepan over medium heat. Add the ham and tomatoes and sauté for 2 to 3 minutes. Add the eggs and spinach and cook, stirring, until the eggs are set. Add the avocado with a pinch of salt and pepper to finish. Serve.

HOMEMADE PARFAIT

SERVES 1

1 1/2 cups 2% Greek yogurt
1 1/2 cups fresh or frozen blueberries
1/2 cup granola (see Jen's specs, page 85)

Combine all the ingredients in a small bowl. Mix well and serve.

NO-BAKE BITES

SERVES 6

1/2 cup almond butter
2 tablespoons unsweetened coconut flakes

1 cup old-fashioned oats (see Jen's specs, page 85), plus more as needed

1 tablespoon jam (any flavor)

1 tablespoon chia seeds

1 tablespoon hemp seeds

1 teaspoon vanilla extract

1/4 cup dark chocolate chips (optional)

In a large bowl, mix together the almond butter, coconut flakes, oats, and jam until well combined. (Use a fork, or even your hands if necessary.) Add the chia seeds, hemp seeds, vanilla, and chocolate chips (if using) and combine. If the mixture is too dry, add a little more almond butter to help it stick together. If it's too wet, add some more oats.

Form the mixture into 12 balls and serve. You can store these in an airtight container in the fridge for up to 1 week, or in the freezer for 1 month.

OATMEAL AND EGG BAKE

SERVES 1

4 egg whites

3/4 cup old-fashioned oats

1 tablespoon peanut butter or almond butter

Ground cinnamon, to taste

Combine the egg whites and oats in a microwave-safe bowl. Microwave for 2 to 3 minutes, or until the egg whites are cooked through. Remove from the microwave. Place the peanut butter on top and allow it to melt. Sprinkle with cinnamon and serve.

OATMEAL GRANOLA COMBO

SERVES 1

1/2 cup cooked oatmeal (or 1/3 cup raw oats)

1/4 cup granola (see Jen's specs, page 85)

1/3 cup berries

1 cup unsweetened almond milk or 2% milk

There are two ways to prepare this breakfast. One is to first cook your oatmeal with water and then transfer it to a small bowl. Sprinkle the granola and berries on top, then add the milk and serve.

The second way is to pour 1/3 cup raw oats, granola, and berries into a small bowl with the milk and eat it like a regular bowl of cereal.

OATMEAL MUFFINS

MAKES 6 MUFFINS (2 MUFFINS PER SERVING)

Vegetable oil cooking spray

1 1/8 cups old-fashioned oats

1/4 cup unsweetened coconut flakes

1/4 teaspoon salt

1/4 teaspoon ground cinnamon

1/4 cup small dried fruit (dried cranberries, dried blueberries, golden raisins, etc.)

2 tablespoons virgin coconut oil, melted and cooled

1 ripe banana, mashed

1 large egg

1 large egg white

Preheat the oven to 350°F. Lightly spray 6 muffin cups with the cooking spray.

In a large bowl, combine the oats, coconut flakes, salt, cinnamon, and dried fruit and mix well. Add the coconut oil, banana, egg, and egg white to the oat mixture and mix completely. The batter will be soft but thick.

Divide the batter evenly among the 6 prepared muffin cups.

Bake for 15 minutes, or until the muffins feel firm when pressed gently in the center.

Remove from the oven and allow to cool in the pan for 10 minutes before serving.

NOTE
You can store these muffins at room temperature for up to 3 days, or put a portion of these in your refrigerator for later in the week.

OPEN-FACED EGG SANDWICH

SERVES 1

1 slice sprouted bread (Ezekiel) or wheat bread, toasted
1/3 avocado, pitted, peeled, and mashed
1 cup fresh spinach
2 eggs plus 2 egg whites, prepared any style
Salt and pepper, to taste

Build the sandwich by topping the bread with each ingredient in order. Serve.

PIZZA OMELET

SERVES 1

Vegetable oil cooking spray
1/2 cup cherry tomatoes, halved
Salt, to taste

Red pepper flakes, to taste
2 large eggs, beaten
2 large egg whites, beaten
1/2 cup shredded mozzarella cheese
Chopped fresh basil

Preheat the oven to 375°F. Spray a small saucepan with the cooking spray.

Add the tomatoes to the prepared pan and sprinkle them with salt and red pepper flakes. Pan-sear the tomatoes over medium heat until they begin to wrinkle and are lightly brown.

Cook the eggs and egg whites in another small, lightly oiled saucepan over medium heat. Once they are set, add the tomatoes, cheese, and basil. Continue to cook over medium heat until the cheese begins to melt. Flip one half of the mixture over to form the omelet. Serve.

PROTEIN OATS 1.0

SERVES 1

1 cup cooked oatmeal
1 scoop protein powder
2 cups fresh berries (any type)

Combine all three ingredients in a small bowl. Mix well and serve.

PROTEIN OATS 2.0

SERVES 1

1 scoop protein powder
1 cup unsweetened vanilla almond milk

1/3 cup old-fashioned oats

1/4 cup granola (see Jen's specs, page 85)

1/2 cup blueberries

In a small bowl, mix the protein powder and almond milk. Stir in the oats, granola, and blueberries. Mix well and serve.

PROTEIN PANCAKES

MAKES 8 PANCAKES (2 PANCAKES PER SERVING)

2 small ripe bananas

2 large eggs

4 large egg whites

2 tablespoons almond or buckwheat flour (optional)

1/4 cup cottage cheese

1/2 teaspoon vanilla extract

1/2 teaspoon ground cinnamon

Vegetable oil cooking spray

In a medium bowl, combine all the ingredients except the cooking spray and whisk until smooth.

Spray a pancake griddle or medium skillet with cooking spray and place it over medium heat. Drop the batter in large spoonfuls onto the griddle. When the batter bubbles, flip the pancakes and brown lightly on the other side. Serve. Store leftover pancakes in the refrigerator.

SCRAMBLED EGG VEGGIE BREAKFAST BURRITO

SERVES 1

2 large eggs

1 large egg white

1/4 teaspoon salt

Pinch of pepper

Vegetable oil cooking spray

Up to 1 cup of any leftover veggies in your fridge from the week

2 tablespoons salsa

1 tortilla (see Jen's specs, page 225)

1/2 avocado, pitted, peeled, and sliced

Hot sauce (optional)

In a small bowl, whisk together the eggs, egg white, salt, and pepper. Heat a nonstick pan over medium-low heat. Lightly spray the pan with the cooking spray. If you're adding leftover veggies, add them to the pan and cook for 2 to 3 minutes, until heated through.

Add the eggs and cook, stirring often, for 3 to 5 minutes, until scrambled. Remove from the heat and gently stir in the salsa.

Place the scrambled egg mixture on a tortilla, add the avocado and some hot sauce (if using), and roll into a burrito to finish. Serve.

STEAK AND EGGS WITH PAN-ROASTED TOMATOES

SERVES 1

6 ounces flank steak

Salt and pepper, to taste

Vegetable oil cooking spray

1 cup cherry tomatoes

2 large eggs

8 to 12 asparagus stalks, ends trimmed

1/2 tablespoon olive oil

Juice of 1/2 lemon

Heat a medium sauté pan over high heat. Sprinkle the steak with a little salt and pepper on both sides. Spray the pan with the cooking spray and add the steak. Reduce the heat to low and cook for 7 to 8 minutes on each side. Add the cherry tomatoes and cook with the steak for about another 2 minutes, until they begin to burst. Transfer the steak and tomatoes to a cutting board and let them rest.

Using the same pan, raise the heat to medium and add a little more cooking spray. Crack the eggs into the pan and cook, sunny side up, for 3 minutes. Sprinkle with salt and pepper.

Thinly slice the steak and transfer it and the tomatoes to a plate with the eggs.

Toss the asparagus with oil, salt, and pepper. Place them under the broiler for 3 to 5 minutes. Remove from the broiler and add to the plate. Drizzle the lemon juice on top to finish. Serve.

VEGGIE SCRAMBLE

SERVES 1

1 large egg, beaten
1 large egg white, beaten
1/4 cup fresh spinach
1/4 cup chopped broccoli
Vegetable oil cooking spray
1/4 avocado, pitted, peeled, and sliced
Salt and pepper, to taste

Mix together the egg, egg white, spinach, and broccoli. Spray a small saucepan with the cooking spray and add the egg mixture. Cook over medium-low heat, stirring often, until the eggs are set and the veggies are tender. Transfer to a plate and top with avocado. Season with salt and pepper and serve.

SMOOTHIES AND SHAKES

3-INGREDIENT SMOOTHIE #1

SERVES 1

1 scoop protein powder (see Jen's specs, page 218)
1 cup strawberries
1 cup whole milk or unsweetened almond milk
Crushed ice, as needed

Place all the ingredients in a blender and blend until smooth. Pour into a glass and serve.

> **JEN JUJU: Super Seeds**
>
> *I've "planted" three amazing seeds on a lot of my recipes for their health benefits. Take a look:*
>
> *Chia seeds, a member of the mint family, are easily digested, are packed with fiber, and can absorb so much water that they make you feel full, plus they help release carbohydrates slowly into your bloodstream for steady energy levels all day. Chia seeds are nutrient-rich, too: just 2 tablespoons provide 8 grams of fiber, 5 grams of protein, 184 milligrams of calcium, and 5 grams of omega-3 fatty acids. You can sprinkle chia seeds over salads and veggies, stir them into yogurt and cereals, and add them to baked goods.*
>
> *Flaxseed provides mucilage fiber, which soothes the intestinal tract and slows down absorption of blood sugar from your intestine, helping to prevent swings in glucose. Mucilage fiber will also keep you regular and ushers bad cholesterol toxins out of your body. And I can't forget to mention flaxseed's other superpowers: it's a source of omega-3 fatty acids, lignans (phytonutrients thought to fight cancer and diabetes), fiber, and proteins. You can use flaxseeds like chia seeds in everything from salads to yogurt to baked goods.*

Hemp seeds are the newer seeds on the block, available in the form of powders, shelled seeds, milk, and oil. A tablespoon of hemp seeds has approximately 11 grams of protein, which is high when compared with a whole egg, which has around 6 grams of protein. Hemp seeds are also packed with essential fatty acids that act like antioxidants in the body, fighting annoying un-wanted free radicals. So hemp up your diet!

3-INGREDIENT SMOOTHIE #2

SERVES 1

1 scoop protein powder (see Jen's specs, page 218)
Large handful of fresh spinach
1 cup whole milk or unsweetened almond milk
Crushed ice, as needed

Place all the ingredients in a blender and blend until smooth. Pour into a glass and serve.

5-INGREDIENT SMOOTHIE

SERVES 1

1 scoop protein powder (see Jen's specs, page 218)
1 cup strawberries
1/4 cup old-fashioned oats (see Jen's specs, page 85)
1 tablespoon chia seeds
1 cup whole milk or unsweetened almond milk
Crushed ice, as needed

Place all the ingredients in a blender and blend until smooth. Pour into a glass and serve.

BANANA BERRY PROTEIN SMOOTHIE

SERVES 1

1½ cups unsweetened vanilla almond milk

1 scoop protein powder (see Jen's specs, page 218)

½ cup old-fashioned oats (see Jen's specs, page 85)

½ cup fresh berries (raspberries, blueberries, or blackberries)

½ banana

1 cup fresh kale

Crushed ice, as needed

Place all the ingredients in a blender and blend until smooth. Pour into a glass and serve.

BANANA NUT PROTEIN SMOOTHIE

SERVES 1

1 cup unsweetened vanilla almond milk or water

1 cup 2% Greek yogurt

¼ cup old-fashioned oats (see Jen's specs, page 85)

1 medium banana

1 tablespoon chia seeds

Crushed ice, as needed

Place all the ingredients in a blender and blend until smooth. Pour into a glass and serve.

BERRIES AND GREENS SMOOTHIE

SERVES 1

1½ cups mixed berries (blueberries, raspberries, and blackberries)

Handful of fresh spinach

Handful of fresh kale

½ cup steamed broccoli florets

1 cup water

Juice of ½ lemon

¼ teaspoon minced fresh ginger (optional)

Crushed ice, as needed

Please all the ingredients in a blender and blend until smooth. Pour into a glass and serve.

BLENDED SHAKE 1.0

SERVES 1

1 scoop protein powder (see Jen's specs, page 218)
2 cups unsweetened vanilla almond milk, 2% milk, or water
1/2 banana
1 tablespoon almond or peanut butter
Handful of fresh kale
Crushed ice, as needed

Place all the ingredients in a blender and blend until smooth. Pour into a glass and serve.

BLENDED SHAKE 2.0

SERVES 1

1/2 cup unsweetened vanilla almond milk or 2% milk
1/2 cup 2% Greek yogurt
1/4 cup old-fashioned oats (see Jen's specs, page 85)
1 cup strawberries
1 cup fresh kale
Crushed ice, as needed

Place all the ingredients in a blender and blend until smooth. Pour into a glass and serve.

BLUEBERRY PROTEIN SMOOTHIE

SERVES 1

1 cup unsweetened vanilla almond milk
1/2 cup water

$1^1/_2$ scoops protein powder (see Jen's specs, below)

1 tablespoon flaxseed

1 cup fresh blueberries

$1^1/_2$ cups fresh spinach

Crushed ice, as needed

Place all the ingredients in a blender and blend until smooth. Pour into a glass and serve.

> **JEN'S SPECS: Protein Powder**
>
> *There are so many protein powders out there that it can be confusing to know which to purchase. My solution is to read the label. Look for a product that supplies 18 to 23 grams of protein, 7 to 10 grams of carbohydrate, and less than 5 grams of sugar per scoop.*

FOREVER YOUNG SMOOTHIE

SERVES 1

1 cup unsweetened vanilla almond milk

$1^1/_2$ scoops protein powder (see Jen's specs, above)

$1^1/_2$ cups fresh kale

$^1/_2$ cup grapefruit sections

$^3/_4$ cup blueberries

$^1/_3$ cup walnuts

Crushed ice, as needed

Place all the ingredients in a blender and blend until smooth. Pour into a glass and serve.

GREEN DETOX SMOOTHIE

1^1/$_2$ cups unsweetened vanilla almond milk
1^1/$_2$ cups fresh spinach
1 cup chopped beets
^{1}/$_2$ banana
^{3}/$_4$ cup chopped cucumber
1 tablespoon flaxseed
Juice of 1 lemon
Crushed ice, as needed

Place all the ingredients in a blender and blend until smooth. Pour into a glass and serve.

GREEN SMOOTHIE

SERVES 1

1 cup water
1 cup fresh spinach
1 cup fresh kale
1 cup chopped cucumber
^{1}/$_2$ Granny Smith apple, peeled, cored, and chopped
^{1}/$_2$ banana
Juice of ^{1}/$_2$ lemon
Large handful of crushed ice

Place all the ingredients in a blender and blend until smooth. Pour into a glass and serve.

GREENS JUICE

SERVES 1

3 celery stalks

1 cucumber

Handful of fresh kale (rolled in a ball in order to better juice)

Handful of fresh spinach (rolled in a ball in order to better juice)

Handful of fresh parsley (rolled in a ball in order to better juice)

1 lemon, quartered

4 large romaine leaves

1 apple, quartered (optional)

1 tablespoon powdered chlorella

1 tablespoon powdered spirulina

Salt, to taste

Juice the celery, cucumber, kale, spinach, parsley, lemon, romaine, and apple (if using) in order according to the juicer manufacturer's instructions. Pour the juice into a tall glass. Stir in the chlorella, spirulina, and salt; mix well. Serve.

PEAR AND MINTED GREENS SMOOTHIE

SERVES 1

1 kiwi

1/2 pear, chopped

Handful of fresh spinach

Handful of fresh kale

1/2 cup steamed broccoli

2 sprigs fresh mint

1 cup water

Juice of 1/2 lemon

¼ teaspoon minced fresh ginger (optional)

Crushed ice, as needed

Place all the ingredients in a blender and blend until smooth. Pour into a glass and serve.

PROTEIN-KALE SMOOTHIE

SERVES 1

1 cup unsweetened vanilla almond milk or water

½ cup coconut water

1 scoop protein powder (see Jen's specs, page 218)

1 tablespoon chia seeds

Handful of fresh kale

Crushed ice, as needed

Place all the ingredients in a blender and blend until smooth. Pour into a glass and serve.

> **JEN JUJU: Drink Your Veggies!**
> *I love to toss vitamin-packed greens like kale and spinach into my smoothies, usually with fruit. You don't even taste the greens, but you get a wallop of their nutrients: vitamins A, C, E, and K, as well as minerals such as calcium, magnesium, zinc, and potassium, plus a bunch of phytonutrients and fiber.*
>
> *Drinking greens in your smoothies is an easy way to increase your daily veggie intake—something we should all be doing but aren't. We can all use more. My favorite smoothie vegetables are spinach and kale, both easily blended into the beverage.*

PROTEIN SMOOTHIE WITH RED BERRIES

SERVES 1

1 cup unsweetened vanilla almond milk or water

1 scoop protein powder (see Jen's specs, page 218)

1/2 cup strawberries

1/2 cup raspberries

1 tablespoon chia seeds

Crushed ice, as needed

Place all the ingredients in a blender and blend until smooth. Pour into a glass and serve.

SIMPLE SHAKE #1

SERVES 1

1 scoop protein powder (see Jen's specs, page 218)

1 tablespoon chia seeds

2 cups unsweetened vanilla almond milk, 2% milk, or water

+Blender bonus: Add 4 ounces fresh or frozen berries with no syrup or added sugar

Crushed ice, as needed

Place all the ingredients in a blender and blend until smooth. Pour into a glass and serve.

SIMPLE SHAKE #2

SERVES 1

1 scoop protein powder (see Jen's specs, page 218)

1 tablespoon almond or peanut butter

2 cups unsweetened vanilla almond milk, 2% milk, or water
Crushed ice, as needed

Place all the ingredients in a blender and blend until smooth. Pour into a glass and serve.

SIMPLE SHAKE #3

SERVES 1

1 scoop protein powder (see Jen's specs, page 218)
2 cups unsweetened vanilla almond milk, 2% milk, or water
+Blender bonus: Add 1/2 banana and a handful of fresh spinach
Crushed ice, as needed

Place all the ingredients in a blender and blend until smooth. Pour into a glass and serve.

SIMPLE SHAKE #4

SERVES 1

1 scoop protein powder (see Jen's specs, page 218)
1 tablespoon chia seeds
2 cups unsweetened vanilla almond milk, 2% milk, or water
+Blender bonus: Add a handful of fresh kale
Crushed ice, as needed

Place all the ingredients in a blender and blend until smooth. Pour into a glass and serve.

STRAWBERRY CHOCOLATE PROTEIN SMOOTHIE

SERVES 1

1 cup unsweetened vanilla almond milk

1 cup 2% Greek yogurt

$1/3$ cup old-fashioned oats (see Jen's specs, page 85)

1 cup strawberries

1 tablespoon chocolate syrup (optional)

Crushed ice, as needed

Place all the ingredients in a blender and blend until smooth. Pour into a glass and serve.

LIGHT LUNCHES

CHICKEN SALAD ROMAINE WRAPS

SERVES 1

1 (5-ounce) can chicken (water packed; organic is best)

2 Persian cucumbers, chopped

2 celery stalks, chopped

2 tablespoons golden raisins

$1^1/_2$ teaspoons extra-virgin olive oil

$1^1/_2$ teaspoons mayonnaise

3 large romaine leaves

1 medium tomato, sliced

Salt and pepper, to taste

In a small bowl, mash together the chicken, cucumbers, celery, raisins, olive oil, and mayonnaise. Place the romaine leaves on a plate. Spread the chicken mixture evenly over the leaves, top with the tomato slices, and season with salt and pepper. Roll up into three wraps and enjoy.

CHICKEN SPINACH SALAD

SERVES 1

4 cups fresh spinach
1/2 cup sliced strawberries
4 to 6 ounces grilled chicken
1/4 cup feta cheese crumbles
Balsamic vinaigrette salad dressing

Arrange the spinach on a plate. Top with the strawberries, chicken, and feta cheese. Drizzle the dressing over the top of the salad. Serve.

CHICKEN WRAP #1

SERVES 1

1 (6-inch) whole-wheat tortilla
5 to 6 ounces grilled chicken
Handful of fresh spinach
1 slice cheese
Handful of bean sprouts

Place the tortilla on a plate. Place the chicken, spinach, cheese, and sprouts on top of the tortilla. Roll up tightly and enjoy.

JEN'S SPECS: Tortillas
Tortillas come in all kinds of crazy forms and colors. It's tough to pick the best type. You can be fooled easily by those bright green or red tortillas, too. Watch it: they're mostly loaded with artificial dyes and not made with veggies.

Here's the deal: pick a wrap with whole-wheat flour listed as the first ingredient. Also, check that 1 serving is actually the whole tortilla, arriving right around 150 calories, 3 to 5 grams of fat, 22 to 26 grams of carbohydrate, 4 to 6 grams of protein, and less than 2 grams of sugar. My favorite brands are Maria and Ricardo's Whole Wheat Tortillas, Trader Joe's Handmade 100% Whole Wheat Flour Tortillas, and Food For Life Ezekiel 4:9 Sprouted Grain Tortillas.

CHICKEN WRAP #2

SERVES 1

1 (6-inch) whole-wheat tortilla

2 tablespoons hummus

5 to 6 ounces grilled chicken

Handful of fresh spinach

3 to 4 slices Persian cucumber

2 tablespoons shredded carrot

Place the tortilla on a plate. Spread the hummus on the tortilla and fill with chicken, spinach, cucumber, and carrot. Roll up tightly and enjoy.

CHICKEN WRAP #3

SERVES 1

1 (6-inch) whole-wheat tortilla

1/3 avocado, pitted, peeled, and sliced

Salt, to taste

5 to 6 ounces grilled chicken

1 to 2 leaves romaine lettuce

1/2 tomato, sliced

Place the tortilla on a plate. Mash the avocado across the tortilla and season lightly with salt. Layer on the chicken, romaine lettuce, and tomato. Roll up tightly and enjoy.

CHOPPED ROMAINE SALAD WITH HERBED VINAIGRETTE

SERVES 1

1/4 head romaine lettuce, chopped

Large handful of fresh spinach

1/2 tomato, chopped

1/2 cucumber, chopped

Fresh corn kernels, sliced off 1 whole cob

1/2 yellow bell pepper, chopped

1/3 cup shredded mozzarella cheese or feta cheese crumbles

FOR THE HERBED VINAIGRETTE

1/4 yellow onion

1 garlic clove

3 tablespoons apple cider vinegar

2 tablespoons fresh lemon or lime juice

Large handful of fresh herbs (use mostly basil and parsley, and if you want, a little mint)

1/4 cup olive oil

1/4 teaspoon cayenne pepper

1/2 teaspoon salt

1/4 teaspoon black pepper

In a small bowl, mix together the romaine, spinach, tomato, cucumber, corn, and bell pepper and set aside.

To make the herbed vinaigrette: Place the onion, garlic, vinegar, lemon juice, herbs, oil, cayenne pepper, salt, and black pepper in a blender and blend until smooth. Pour the vinaigrette over the salad, just enough to coat, and toss. Store any remaining dressing in the fridge. Transfer to a plate and top with the cheese to serve.

CREAMY BUTTERNUT SQUASH SOUP

SERVES 2

1 tablespoon olive oil

1/2 medium butternut squash, peeled, seeded, and cubed (1 to 2 cups) (see Notes)

1/2 yellow onion, chopped

1 garlic clove

1 teaspoon salt, plus more to taste

3/4 cup unsweetened almond or coconut milk

Heat a large skillet over medium-high heat. Add the olive oil, squash, onion, garlic, and 1 teaspoon salt and sauté for 12 to 15 minutes, until the squash is lightly browned and cooked through.

Place the squash in a blender (see Notes), add the milk, and blend until very smooth, 1 to 2 minutes. Ladle into a bowl, season with salt to taste, and serve.

NOTES

You can also buy precut butternut squash.

When using a blender with hot liquid, do not fill it all the way. Place the top of the blender on, vent the lid, and cover with a kitchen towel to allow steam to escape.

This soup freezes great! Or you can keep leftovers in the fridge for later in the week.

EGG SALAD

SERVES 1

3 hard-boiled eggs, shells removed, chopped (use 2 yolks only; discard the third)

2 celery stalks, chopped

1 pickle spear, minced (optional)

1^1/$_2$ teaspoons olive oil or mayonnaise

1 to 2 teaspoons mustard (any type)

Salt and pepper, to taste

2 to 3 cups leafy greens, or leaves for wrapping

In a small bowl, mix the eggs, celery, pickle (if using), oil, mustard, salt, and pepper. Place the leafy greens on a plate, top with the egg salad, and wrap up. Serve.

GRILLED TUNA WITH BROWN RICE AND VEGGIES

SERVES 1

1 (6-ounce) tuna steak

1 tablespoon olive oil, plus more for brushing

Salt and pepper, to taste

1 to 2 cups snap peas

Juice of 1 lemon

1 cup cooked brown rice

Heat a grill or indoor grill pan to high heat. Brush the tuna with olive oil and sprinkle with salt and pepper. Place the tuna on the grill and cook for 2^1/$_2$ to 3^1/$_2$ minutes on each side, until seared on the outside and pink in the middle. Remove from the grill and let rest for 5 minutes.

Bring a small pot of water to a boil. Once boiling, add a large pinch of salt. Add the snap peas and cook for 1 to 2 minutes, until bright green. Drain. Place the snap peas in a bowl of ice water for 1 minute to stop the cooking. Drain again, transfer to a plate, and top with half the lemon juice and a dash of salt.

In a small bowl, mix the cooked brown rice with the 1 tablespoon olive oil, the remaining lemon juice, and a pinch of salt.

Add the rice and tuna to the plate with the snap peas and serve.

HEARTY MINESTRONE SOUP

SERVES 3

1 tablespoon olive oil

1 small yellow onion, chopped

1 cup diced carrots

1 cup diced celery

1 cup diced zucchini

2 garlic cloves, minced

1 teaspoon minced fresh thyme

1 (14-ounce) can chopped tomatoes

3 to 4 cups chicken stock

1 bay leaf

1½ teaspoons salt, plus more to taste

½ teaspoon pepper

½ can white beans, drained and rinsed

2 to 3 large handfuls of fresh baby spinach

2 tablespoons fresh lemon juice

In a large pan, heat the oil over medium heat. Add the onion, carrots, and celery and cook for 8 to 10 minutes, until the veggies begin to soften. Add the zucchini, garlic, and thyme and cook for another 3 to 5 minutes.

Add the tomatoes, 3 cups of the stock, the bay leaf, 1½ teaspoons salt, and the pepper and stir to combine. Bring the soup to a boil, then reduce the heat and simmer uncovered for 20 minutes.

Discard the bay leaf. Add the beans and heat through. Add more stock if needed.

Just before serving, add the spinach and stir until wilted. Stir in the lemon juice and add salt to taste.

Ladle into a bowl and serve.

HIGH-PROTEIN PITA POCKET

SERVES 1

1 (5-ounce) can cooked salmon (or use leftovers) (Jen's salmon specs: Look for skinless, boneless, and naturally 97% fat-free, wild caught)

1/3 cup 2% Greek yogurt

Chopped fresh dill, to taste

2 cups mixed greens

1 slice pita bread

In a small bowl, mix the salmon, yogurt, and dill. Fold in the greens. Place the pita slice on a plate and stuff it with the salmon mixture. Serve.

KALE AND ROMAINE CHOP

SERVES 1

1 cup chopped romaine lettuce

1 cup chopped fresh kale

1/2 cucumber, chopped

1 beet, cooked and chopped

1 cup chopped broccoli

1/3 cup shredded carrot

1 cup shaved Brussels sprouts

1 tablespoon sunflower seeds

1/2 avocado, pitted, peeled, and diced, or 1 ounce shredded cheese (any type) (optional)

Bottled salad dressing, low-calorie/ low sugar

In a medium bowl, combine the romaine, kale, cucumber, beet, broccoli, carrot, Brussels sprouts, sunflower seeds, and avocado or cheese (if using) and mix well. Transfer to a plate and serve with the salad dressing on the side. Dip your fork into the dressing, then spear your salad for each bite.

THE KALE SALAD

2 cups chopped romaine lettuce

2 cups chopped fresh kale

1/4 cup shaved or shredded Parmesan

1/4 cup golden raisins

1/2 cup cooked red or regular quinoa

1/4 cup slivered almonds

4 to 6 ounces diced grilled chicken or vegetarian protein, or
    2 hard-boiled eggs, shells removed, chopped (optional)

Juice of 1/2 lemon

1 tablespoon olive oil

In a medium bowl, combine the romaine, kale, Parmesan, raisins, quinoa, almonds, and chicken or eggs (if using) and mix well. In a small bowl, combine the lemon juice and olive oil. Drizzle the lemon-juice-and-oil blend over the salad to slightly coat it. Transfer to a plate and serve.

MEDITERRANEAN ROMAINE WRAPS

4 large romaine leaves

3 to 4 tablespoons hummus

8 ounces grilled or baked chicken, cut into strips or cubes

1 medium tomato, sliced and salted

3 Persian cucumbers, sliced

2 tablespoons chopped olives (any kind)

2 tablespoons feta cheese crumbles

Place the romaine leaves on a plate and spread with the hummus. Layer the chicken, tomato, and cucumbers on each leaf. Top with olives and feta cheese. Roll up tightly to create a lettuce wrap and serve.

MISO SEAWEED DETOX BROTH

MAKES 15 CUPS (1 CUP PER SERVING);
NOTE: NEED 3 HOURS TO PREP AND COOK

2 packages dried seaweed (wakame or arame is great for
    soups)

15 cups cold filtered water

4 large carrots, roughly chopped

1 cup roughly chopped leek (white and green parts)

1 onion, roughly chopped

1 tablespoon sea salt, or to taste

$1^1/_2$-inch piece fresh ginger

4 heaping tablespoons white miso

In a large bowl of tap water, soak the seaweed for 2 hours or until soft. Drain and rinse well, as dried seaweed can come with a lot of dirt.

Place the seaweed, filtered water, carrots, leek, onion, sea salt, and ginger in a large pot and bring to a boil. Reduce the heat to low and simmer for 30 minutes. Add the miso and stir to combine. Let simmer for another couple of minutes, then strain the broth.

Ladle 1 cup into a bowl and serve. The rest can be stored in an airtight container in the refrigerator for the duration of Phase 1.

OPEN-FACED DELI SAMMY

SERVES 1

1 slice sprouted bread

2 tablespoons hummus

4 to 6 ounces sliced deli meat (Jen's specs: prioritize organic,
    nitrate-free brands)

Several fresh spinach leaves

2 tomato slices

Place the bread on a plate and spread it with the hummus. Top with the deli meat, spinach, and tomato. Serve open-faced.

ROASTED SWEET POTATO AND CAULIFLOWER SOUP

SERVES 2

2 medium sweet potatoes, cubed

2 cups cauliflower florets

1/4 cup sliced shallots

1 garlic clove

1 tablespoon olive oil

1/2 teaspoon salt, plus more to taste

1/4 teaspoon pepper, plus more to taste

1 1/2 to 2 cups chicken or vegetable stock

Toasted sunflower seeds, for garnish

Preheat the oven to 400°F.

Place the sweet potatoes, cauliflower, shallots, and garlic on a sheet pan. Toss with the olive oil, 1/2 teaspoon salt, and 1/4 teaspoon pepper until well coated. Roast for 30 to 35 minutes, until the veggies are soft and begin to caramelize. Remove from the oven and set aside.

In batches, pour the veggie mixture and stock into a blender (see Notes) and blend until smooth and creamy, about 1 minute, or to your desired texture. I add 1 to 2 cups veggies with 1 cup stock to start, and adjust accordingly. For a thinner soup, add more stock.

Pour each batch of veggie purée into a medium pot and repeat until all the veggies have been blended. Once the entire soup is puréed, add the salt and pepper to taste. (I add about another 1/2 teaspoon salt.)

Heat through over medium-low heat until hot. Ladle into a bowl and finish with a sprinkle of toasted sunflower seeds before serving.

NOTES

When using a blender with hot liquid, do not fill it all the way. Place the top of the blender on, vent the lid, and cover with a kitchen towel to allow the steam to escape.

This soup freezes great!

ROASTED VEGETABLE SALAD

SERVES 1

1 cup diced butternut squash (cut into 1-inch pieces)
2 cups cauliflower florets, broken into pieces
1 cup mushrooms, cleaned and stems removed
2 tablespoons extra-virgin olive oil
Salt and pepper, to taste
1/2 cup cherry tomatoes, halved
1/2 avocado, pitted, peeled, and diced
1/4 cup dried cranberries
3 cups arugula

Preheat the oven to 425°F.

Evenly place the squash, cauliflower, and mushrooms on a baking sheet and drizzle the veggies with the oil. Season with salt and pepper.

Roast for 25 to 30 minutes, or until the veggies are golden brown. Remove from the oven and allow to cool. Then toss the roasted vegetables with the tomatoes, avocado, and cranberries. Place the arugula on a plate and top with the veggie mixture. Serve.

SALMON BURGERS ON BUTTER LETTUCE

SERVES 1

6 ounces salmon, cut into small pieces
1 bundle green onions (scallions), white and green parts, chopped
Sea salt and pepper, to taste
Juice of 1/2 lemon
2 tablespoons olive oil
Vegetable oil cooking spray
Butter lettuce leaves

In a small bowl, mix the salmon, onion, salt, pepper, lemon juice, and olive oil and form the mixture into mini patties.

Spray a skillet with the cooking spray. Add the patties and cook over medium-high heat, 2 to 3 minutes on each side. Place the butter lettuce leaves on a plate, top with the burgers, and serve.

NOTE
This dish travels well! It can be eaten hot or cold or reheated.

SANDWICH WRAP

1 wheat or rice tortilla

Large handful of fresh spinach leaves

1 cup bean sprouts

2 to 3 tomato slices

1 ounce cheese (any type)

6 to 8 ounces protein (optional)

Place the tortilla on a plate and top it with the spinach, bean sprouts, tomato, and cheese. If desired, you can add meat—for example, grilled chicken, organic deli chicken, or Applegate Farms turkey. Roll up the tortilla tightly to create a wrap. Serve.

SEARED AHI TUNA SALAD

SERVES 1

2 cups mixed greens

6 ounces cooked sushi-grade tuna

Soy sauce, to taste

2 teaspoons sesame seeds

2 tablespoons chopped green onion (scallions)

Arrange the greens on a plate. Top with the tuna. Drizzle soy sauce over the tuna and greens. Sprinkle with the sesame seeds and scallion. Serve.

SHAVED BRUSSELS SPROUTS SALAD

SERVES 1

8 ounces shaved or thinly sliced Brussels sprouts (about 3 cups)
1/2 cup cooked black rice
1/2 cup cashews
5 pitted dates, thinly sliced
1/4 cup pomegranate seeds

FOR THE DRESSING
2 tablespoons fresh lemon juice
2 tablespoons olive oil
2 teaspoons capers

In a medium bowl, combine the Brussels sprouts, rice, cashews, dates, and pomegranate seeds and mix together.

To make the dressing: Whisk together the lemon juice, oil, and capers. Add the dressing to the salad and toss well. Transfer to a plate and serve.

NOTE
This dish can be served chilled or at room temperature.

SOUTHWEST VEGGIE CHOP

SERVES 1

1/4 head romaine lettuce, chopped
Handful of chopped fresh spinach
1/2 cup diced tomato
1 cup diced cucumber
1 cup diced red bell pepper
1 cup black beans
1/2 cup fresh corn kernels, sliced off the cob

¼ cup shredded mozzarella cheese

Balsamic vinegar, for drizzling

Place the lettuce and spinach in a salad bowl and set aside. Add the tomato, cucumber, bell pepper, beans, corn, and cheese and toss well. Drizzle with balsamic vinegar and serve.

SPINACH AND PEAR SALAD

SERVES 1

6 cups fresh spinach

1 pear, sliced

1 cup cottage cheese

2 tablespoons diced red onion

1 tablespoon toasted pine nuts

6 to 8 ounces protein (optional)

Arrange the spinach on a plate. Top with the pear slices, followed by the cottage cheese, onion, and nuts. Serve with other protein, if desired.

STRENGTHENING BONE BROTH

MAKES 16 CUPS (1 CUP PER SERVING);
NOTE: NEED 11+ HOURS TO PREPARE AND COOK

2 pounds grass-fed marrow bones

2 tablespoons organic apple cider vinegar, such as Bragg's

1 head garlic

10 to 12 whole cloves

1 teaspoon sea salt, or to taste

1 gallon filtered water

Place all the ingredients in a slow cooker. If desired, brown the marrow bones in a pan first to add flavor. Cook on high until the broth boils; then reduce the heat to low and cook for an additional 10 to 24 hours. (The longer, the better.) Let the broth cool, then strain and discard the solids. Ladle into a bowl and serve. You can store the rest in lidded glass jars in the fridge for a few days. Alternatively, freeze it if you need to store it longer.

TUNA SALAD

SERVES 1

2 to 3 cups leafy greens

1 (5-ounce) can tuna (water packed), drained, or 5 ounces diced cooked chicken breast

1/2 Granny Smith apple, chopped

2 celery stalks, chopped

1 1/2 teaspoons olive oil

2 tablespoons white wine vinegar

1 to 2 teaspoons mustard (any type), to taste

1/2 cup cherry tomatoes (optional)

1/4 cup shaved Parmesan (optional)

Arrange the greens on a plate. In a small bowl, combine the remaining ingredients, place on the greens, and serve.

TUNA SALAD WRAPS

SERVES 1

1 (5-ounce) can tuna (water packed), drained, or 5 ounces diced cooked chicken breast

1/2 cup chopped apple

2 celery stalks, chopped

1½ teaspoons olive oil

2 tablespoons white wine vinegar

1 to 2 teaspoons mustard

2 to 3 romaine leaves

2 to 3 tomato slices

2 to 3 cheese slices

In a small bowl, combine the tuna, apple, celery, oil, vinegar, and mustard. Place the romaine leaves on a plate and divide the tuna salad among the leaves. Top each with a tomato slice and a cheese slice. Roll up the leaves and enjoy.

TURMERIC LENTIL AND FARRO SOUP

SERVES 2

1 tablespoon olive oil

½ small onion, grated (about ½ cup)

1 small zucchini, grated (about 1 cup)

½ cup grated carrot

¾ teaspoon salt

¼ teaspoon pepper

¾ teaspoon turmeric

¼ teaspoon ground cumin

2½ cups vegetable or chicken broth

¼ cup quick-cooking farro (I use the 10-minute farro from Trader Joe's)

¼ cup red lentils

¾ cup chopped fresh kale or chopped fresh spinach

In a medium pot, heat the oil over medium-high heat. Add the onion, zucchini, and carrot and cook for 1 to 2 minutes. Add the salt, pepper, turmeric, and cumin and cook for another 2 to 3 minutes. You should start to smell the spices toasting.

Stir in the broth and bring to a boil. Once boiling, add the farro and lentils and simmer over low heat for 15 to 20 minutes, or until the farro and lentils are cooked through.

In the last few minutes of cooking, add the kale and stir until wilted. Ladle into a bowl and serve.

EVERYDAY ENTRÉES

BAKED GARLIC-LEMON SALMON WITH HERBED BROWN RICE AND ASPARAGUS

SERVES 1

Vegetable oil cooking spray

5 ounces salmon

1 teaspoon olive oil

1/4 teaspoon salt

1/4 teaspoon pepper

1 garlic clove, minced

1 lemon

FOR THE HERBED BROWN RICE

1 cup cooked brown rice (Trader Joe's makes a great quick and easy frozen brown rice)

1 teaspoon olive oil

Pinch of salt

1 tablespoon chopped cilantro (or any herbs you love!)

FOR THE ASPARAGUS

8 ounces asparagus stalks, ends trimmed

1 teaspoon olive oil

1/4 teaspoon salt

1/4 teaspoon pepper

1/4 teaspoon garlic powder

1 lemon

Preheat the oven to 375°F. Spray a baking dish with the cooking spray.

In the prepared dish, brush the salmon with the olive oil, and sprinkle evenly with the salt, pepper, and garlic. Cut two thin slices of lemon and place them on top of the salmon.

Bake for 20 to 25 minutes, until the fish is flaky. Remove from the oven, transfer to a plate, and squeeze juice from half the remaining lemon over the top to finish.

To make the herbed brown rice: In a bowl, combine the rice, oil, salt, and cilantro. Use a fork to combine well. Transfer to the plate with the fish.

To make the asparagus: Preheat the broiler. Place the asparagus on a sheet pan and toss with the olive oil, salt, pepper, and garlic powder. Broil for about 5 minutes, until lightly browned and tender-crisp. Remove from the broiler, transfer to the plate with the fish and rice, and squeeze juice from the remaining lemon half over the top to finish. Serve.

BAKED SESAME SALMON WITH ROASTED VEGGIES

SERVES 1

Vegetable oil cooking spray

6 ounces salmon

2 tablespoons olive oil, plus more for brushing the salmon

Salt and pepper, to taste

1/2 teaspoon garlic powder

2 tablespoons soy sauce

1 cup cauliflower florets

1 cup diced or baby carrots

2 tablespoons toasted sesame seeds

Preheat the oven to 400°F. Spray a baking dish with the cooking spray.

Place the salmon in the prepared dish, brush it with oil, and sprinkle lightly with the salt, pepper, and garlic powder. Pour the soy sauce over the salmon. Set aside.

On a sheet pan, toss the cauliflower and carrots with the 2 table-spoons oil and a large pinch of salt and pepper.

Bake everything together in the oven for 20 to 25 minutes. Remove from the oven, transfer to a plate, and sprinkle with the toasted sesame seeds to finish. Serve.

BAKED WHITEFISH WITH OVEN-ROASTED VEGGIES

SERVES 1

Vegetable oil cooking spray
5 ounces whitefish
2 teaspoons olive oil
$1/2$ teaspoon salt
$1/2$ teaspoon lemon pepper
1 lemon

FOR THE OVEN-ROASTED VEGGIES

1 cup cauliflower florets
1 cup halved Brussels sprouts
2 tablespoons olive oil
$1/2$ teaspoon salt
$1/4$ teaspoon black pepper
$1/4$ teaspoon garlic powder

Preheat the oven to 350°F. Spray a baking dish with the cooking spray.

Place the fish in the prepared dish. Brush the fish lightly with the oil and sprinkle with 1/4 teaspoon of the salt and 1/4 teaspoon of the lemon pepper. Turn the fish over and repeat on the other side with the remaining 1/2 teaspoon salt and 1/2 teaspoon lemon pepper.

Place 1 or 2 thin slices of lemon on top of the fish and bake for 20 to 25 minutes until the fish is flaky and cooked through. Remove from the oven, transfer to a plate, and squeeze the juice of the remaining lemon over the top to finish.

To make the oven-roasted veggies (see Notes): Place the cauliflower and Brussels sprouts in a single layer on a large sheet pan. Toss with the oil, salt, black pepper, and garlic powder. Roast for 30 to 35 minutes until slightly browned and tender. Stir the veggies halfway through the cooking time. Remove from the oven and transfer to the plate with the fish. Serve.

NOTES
Fish and veggies can cook in the oven at the same time.

Veggies can also be made ahead of time and stored in the fridge.

BBQ BAKED CHICKEN

SERVES 1

1 tablespoon melted butter
3 tablespoons barbecue sauce
1 (6- to 8-ounce) boneless skinless chicken breast
Vegetable oil cooking spray
2 cups broccoli florets
1/2 cup chickpeas, rinsed and drained
1 1/2 teaspoons olive oil
1 teaspoon salt
1 teaspoon garlic powder

Preheat the oven to 425°F.

In a small bowl, combine the butter and barbecue sauce. Place the chicken breast in a small glass baking dish and brush it with the sauce on both sides.

Bake for 15 to 18 minutes, until cooked through.

Remove from the oven, cover lightly with foil, and let rest for 10 minutes.

Line a baking sheet with foil and spray with the cooking spray. Add the broccoli and chickpeas and toss with the olive oil, salt, and garlic powder until well coated.

Bake for 15 to 20 minutes until the broccoli is cooked through and the chickpeas begin to crisp. Remove from the oven. Transfer the chicken, broccoli, and chickpeas to a plate and serve.

BISON BAKE

SERVES 1

Vegetable oil cooking spray
2 cups fresh baby kale
1 (5-ounce) bison patty
5 ounces cubed sweet potato
3/4 cup broccoli
3/4 cup cauliflower
1 tablespoon olive oil
1/2 teaspoon salt
1/4 teaspoon pepper
1/4 teaspoon ground cumin

Preheat the oven to 400°F. Spray a glass baking dish with the cooking spray.

Place the kale in the bottom of the prepared dish and top with the bison patty. Toss the sweet potato, broccoli, and cauliflower with the olive oil, salt, pepper, and cumin. Add the veggies to the baking dish and bake for 20 to 25 minutes, or until vegetables are tender and the bison patty is cooked to your liking. Remove from the oven, transfer to a plate, and serve.

BISON BEEF MEATBALLS WITH BAKED SWEET POTATO

SERVES 1

FOR THE BAKED SWEET POTATO

1 medium sweet potato
Salt and pepper, to taste

FOR THE BISON BEEF MEATBALLS

1/4 pound onion, peeled and finely chopped
2 garlic cloves, minced
1/2 pound ground bison or 93% lean turkey meat
1/4 teaspoon sea salt
1 teaspoon black pepper
1/2 teaspoon low-sodium soy sauce
1 teaspoon dried oregano
1 tablespoon chopped fresh sage
Pinch of cayenne pepper
1/2 cup panko bread crumbs
1 large egg, beaten
1 1/2 teaspoons extra-virgin olive oil

To make the baked sweet potato: Preheat the oven to 400°F. Using a fork, prick some holes all over the sweet potato. Wrap in foil and bake for 45 to 55 minutes, until a knife is easily inserted into the center. Remove from the oven, slice the potato open, and sprinkle with the salt and pepper. (See Note for microwave option.)

To make the bison beef meatballs: In a medium bowl, combine the onion, garlic, bison, salt, black pepper, soy sauce, oregano, sage, cayenne pepper, panko, and egg. Mix well without overworking, which can create a heavy paste. Form the mixture into 6 meatballs. In a saucepan over medium heat, brown the meatballs in the oil on all sides, 5 to 10 minutes.

Transfer the meatballs and potato to a plate and serve.

NOTE
To cook a sweet potato in the microwave, simply prick some holes all over the sweet potato, wrap it in a wet paper towel, place in the microwave on a microwave safe-dish, and cook for 5 to 7 minutes, or until soft. DO NOT USE FOIL IN THE MICROWAVE!

BISON MEATBALLS AND ROASTED SPAGHETTI SQUASH

SERVES 2

3/4 pound ground bison
1 tablespoon chopped fresh sage
1 tablespoon chopped fresh parsley
1/4 cup chopped green onions (scallions), green parts only
1/4 teaspoon paprika
Salt and pepper, to taste
1 tablespoon extra-virgin olive oil
1 spaghetti squash
1 (13-ounce) jar low-sugar and/or low-carb marinara sauce

Preheat the oven to 400°F.

In a medium bowl, combine the bison, sage, parsley, scallions, paprika, salt, and pepper and form into golf-ball-size meatballs. In a large pan, heat the oil over medium-high heat. Add the meatballs and cook for 2 to 3 minutes on every side (this should take 8 to 10 minutes).

Cut the squash lengthwise and remove and discard the seeds. Place the squash halves cut side down in a baking dish, add 1/4 cup water, cover with foil, and bake for 45 minutes. Don't let the water cook away; check it during baking and add more if needed. Remove from the oven and allow the squash to cool slightly, then scrape out the strands with a fork and transfer to a plate.

Heat the marinara sauce. Serve the meatballs over the squash and top with the marinara sauce.

BREAKFAST FOR DINNER

SERVES 1

2 bacon strips or 2 turkey links or patties
1 bell pepper (any color), thinly sliced
1 small yellow onion, sliced
Salt and pepper, to taste
2 large eggs

Lay the bacon strips in a cold nonstick pan. Turn the heat on low and cook to the desired crispiness. Remove the bacon from the pan and lay it on a paper-towel-lined plate.

Drain any excess fat and use the same pan to cook the veggies and eggs. Don't wash the pan in between! The leftover bacon flavor will help make your veggies and eggs awesome! Heat the pan over medium-high heat. Add the bell pepper, onion, and a pinch of salt and pepper. Cook for about 10 minutes, until soft. Remove from the pan and set aside on a plate.

In a small bowl, whisk the eggs with a pinch of salt and pepper. Heat the pan over medium-low heat. Add the eggs and cook until scrambled, stirring often, 3 to 5 minutes. Transfer to the plate with the veggies, add the bacon, and serve.

BURGER BAKE

SERVES 1

Vegetable oil cooking spray
4 ounces 90% lean ground beef
1/2 teaspoon salt
1/4 teaspoon pepper
1/2 teaspoon garlic powder
1/4 teaspoon dried oregano
1 garlic clove, minced
2 cups fresh baby kale
5 ounces sweet potato, cubed
1 cup Brussels sprouts

Preheat the oven to 400°F. Spray a glass baking dish with the cooking spray.

In a bowl, gently mix the beef, salt, pepper, garlic powder, oregano, and garlic, then form into a patty. Arrange the kale, sweet potato, and Brussels sprouts in the prepared baking dish, and place the beef patty on top. Bake for 20 to 25 minutes, or until vegetables are tender and the beef patty is cooked through to your liking. Remove from the oven, transfer to a plate, and serve.

BURGER BOWL

SERVES 1

Vegetable oil cooking spray
6 to 8 ounces 90% lean ground beef or 93% lean ground turkey
3 to 4 cups romaine and/or spinach leaves, chopped
1 slice cheese (any type)
1 tomato slice
1 dill pickle, chopped

Handful of fresh mushrooms

1/4 cup chopped onion

Spray a skillet with the cooking spray. Brown the meat in the skillet over medium-high heat until done. Drain. Place the lettuce leaves on a plate or in a bowl. Top with the meat, cheese, tomato, pickle, mushrooms, and onion. Serve.

BURGER PATTY WITH VEGGIE QUINOA SALAD

SERVES 1

FOR THE BURGER PATTY

1 (6-ounce) beef patty, store-bought or homemade (see Note)

1/2 teaspoon salt

1/4 teaspoon pepper

1/2 teaspoon garlic powder

1/4 teaspoon onion powder

1/4 teaspoon paprika

Vegetable oil cooking spray

FOR THE VEGGIE QUINOA SALAD

1 cup cooked quinoa

1/4 cup quartered cherry tomatoes

1/4 cup diced red onion

1/4 cup diced cucumber

1 tablespoon chopped fresh mint

2 tablespoons olive oil

2 tablespoons red wine vinegar

2 tablespoons fresh lemon juice

Salt, to taste

2 cups fresh spinach

To make the burger patty: Sprinkle the beef patty evenly on both sides with salt, pepper, garlic powder, onion powder, and paprika. Heat a nonstick skillet over medium-high heat. Lightly spray the skillet with the cooking spray and add the beef patty. Cook for 5 to 7 minutes per inch of thickness on each side. Remove from the pan and let rest for 3 to 5 minutes.

To make the veggie quinoa salad: In a large bowl, combine the quinoa, tomatoes, onion, cucumber, and mint.

In a separate bowl, whisk together the oil, vinegar, 1 tablespoon lemon juice, and the salt until combined. Pour the dressing over the quinoa and toss to combine.

To finish, place the spinach on a plate, drizzle with the remaining 1 tablespoon lemon juice, and top with the quinoa and burger.

NOTE
To make a homemade beef patty, you will need 5 ounces ground beef. In a bowl, use a fork to combine the meat and spices. Use your hands to form the meat into a patty and cook according to the directions.

BUTTER LETTUCE FISH TACOS WITH SPICY APPLE SLAW

SERVES 1

FOR THE BUTTER LETTUCE FISH TACOS

Vegetable oil cooking spray

6 to 8 ounces whitefish

6 butter lettuce leaves

1/2 avocado, pitted, peeled, and mashed

FOR THE SPICY APPLE SLAW

1/2 apple, chopped

1 cup shredded cabbage

1 bundle green onions (scallions), white and green parts, chopped

2 tablespoons fresh lemon juice

2 tablespoons fresh lime juice

1 tablespoon olive oil

Sea salt, to taste

Garlic powder, to taste

Chipotle pepper, to taste

To make the butter lettuce fish tacos: Spray a small skillet with the cooking spray. Add the fish and sauté over medium heat, covered, for about 3 minutes on each side.

Meanwhile, to make the spicy apple slaw: In a small bowl, mix together the apple, cabbage, and scallions. Set aside.

To make the dressing: In a small bowl, mix together all the ingredients.

Toss the apple slaw with the dressing. Refrigerate for a short while to let the flavors mingle.

Double the lettuce leaves on a plate to create three taco wrappers. Spread the leaves with the mashed avocado. Fill the leaves with the fish and slaw (or serve on the side), roll up tightly, and serve.

CRANBERRY NUT KALE SALAD

SERVES 1

4 to 5 cups finely chopped fresh kale

1/2 cup toasted pecans, roughly chopped

2 tablespoons toasted pine nuts

2 tablespoons dried cranberries

1/4 yellow onion

1 garlic clove

3 tablespoons apple cider vinegar

2 tablespoons lemon or lime juice

Large handful of fresh herbs (I use mostly parsley, basil, and a little thyme and mint)

¹/₄ cup olive oil

¹/₄ teaspoon cayenne pepper

¹/₂ teaspoon salt

¹/₄ teaspoon black pepper

In a large bowl, combine the kale, pecans, pine nuts, and cranberries. Set aside.

Place the onion, garlic, vinegar, lemon juice, herbs, oil, cayenne pepper, salt, and black pepper in a blender and blend until smooth. Pour the dressing over the salad, just enough to coat. Toss to combine, transfer to a plate, and serve. Store any remaining dressing in the fridge.

DIY STIR-FRY

SERVES 1

1 tablespoon olive oil, plus more as needed

6 to 8 ounces protein (organic tofu, soy and nondairy products acceptable)

2 to 3 cups mixed Asian vegetables, such as broccoli, onions, watercress, shredded carrot, and bok choy

Low-sodium soy sauce

Hot sauce (optional)

Coat a skillet or wok with oil. Add the protein and cook through over medium-high heat. (Shrimp will take no longer than 3 minutes.) Remove from the heat and transfer to a plate.

Add the vegetables to the skillet and cook over medium-high heat until just tender. Add more oil if necessary.

Reduce the temperature to low, add the protein, and heat thoroughly. Transfer to a plate, season with the soy sauce and hot sauce (if using), and serve.

EGGPLANT PARMESAN

SERVES 2

Vegetable oil cooking spray
1 small eggplant
Salt, to taste
2 tablespoons olive oil
Pepper, to taste
1 cup marinara sauce
1/2 cup shredded mozzarella cheese
1/2 cup grated Parmesan cheese
2 tablespoons chopped fresh basil

Preheat the oven to 400°F. Spray a baking dish with the cooking spray.

Peel the eggplant (if desired) and slice it into 1/4-inch slices. Salt the eggplant slices and let them drain in a colander for about 20 minutes. This will remove most of the bitterness. Once the eggplant has released its water, rinse and pat dry.

Place the eggplant in a single layer in the prepared baking dish. Brush the eggplant with the oil and sprinkle with the salt and pepper. Bake for 20 to 30 minutes, or until the eggplant is tender.

Remove from the oven and evenly spoon the marinara sauce on top of the eggplant slices. Sprinkle evenly with mozzarella and Parmesan and place back in the oven for another 10 minutes, or until the cheese is melted and bubbly. Remove from the oven and finish with the chopped basil.

Transfer to a plate and serve.

FARM TO SEA STIR-FRY

SERVES 1

6 to 8 ounces shrimp, peeled and deveined (you can buy them
 this way)

2 tablespoons olive oil

Pinch of lemon pepper

Salt

Pinch of black pepper

2 cups chopped squash (butternut or kabocha)

2 cups chopped zucchini

1 cup snap peas

In a small bowl, toss the shrimp with 1 tablespoon of the oil and a
pinch of lemon pepper and salt. Set aside.

Heat a large pan over medium heat. Add the remaining 1 tablespoon
oil and the squash. Sprinkle with salt and black pepper and cook for
10 to 12 minutes, until cooked through. Add the zucchini and snap
peas to the pan in the last 3 to 5 minutes of cooking. Remove the veggies from the pan and set aside.

Add the shrimp to the pan. Cook for 2 minutes on each side until they
begin to curl. Remove from the heat, return the veggies to the pan,
and toss together.

Transfer to a plate and serve.

FISH STEW

SERVES 2

4 tablespoons olive oil

1 small onion, chopped

2 to 3 garlic cloves, chopped

1 medium tomato, chopped

2 teaspoons tomato paste

1 cup clam juice

1/2 cup dry white wine

1 pound fresh halibut fillets (or red snapper, sole, or sea bass), cut in 2-inch pieces

1/4 cup chopped fresh parsley

1/4 teaspoon dried oregano

1/4 teaspoon black pepper

Dash of Tabasco sauce, or to taste

Heat the oil in a large, heavy pot over medium-high heat. Add the onion and sauté for 2 to 3 minutes, until translucent.

Add the garlic and cook for 1 more minute. Add the tomato and tomato paste and cook over medium-low heat for about 10 minutes.

Add the clam juice, white wine, and fish and simmer for about another 10 minutes, or until the fish is cooked through. Add the parsley, oregano, pepper, and Tabasco sauce and stir to combine.

Transfer to a plate and serve.

FOIL-WRAPPED FISH 1.0

SERVES 1

6 ounces whitefish, such as sole, trout, or orange roughy

1 cup chopped fresh kale

1/2 cup chopped red bell pepper

Juice of 1/2 lemon

Salt and pepper, to taste

1 teaspoon olive oil

Preheat the oven to 400°F.

Place the fish on a large piece of aluminum foil and top with the kale, bell pepper, and lemon juice. Season with salt and pepper and drizzle with the oil. Fold the foil up to tightly seal the ingredients.

Bake for 15 to 20 minutes, or until the fish flakes easily with a fork. Remove from the oven and unwrap from the foil. Transfer to a plate and serve.

FOIL-WRAPPED FISH 2.0

SERVES 1

6 ounces salmon

2 slices lemon

1/2 cup cherry tomatoes, halved

1/2 onion, sliced

8 to 10 asparagus stalks, ends trimmed

Salt and pepper, to taste

1 teaspoon olive oil

Preheat the oven to 400°F.

Place the fish on a large piece of aluminum foil and top with the lemon slices. Layer on the tomatoes, onion, and asparagus. Season with salt and pepper and drizzle with the olive oil. Fold the foil up to tightly seal the ingredients.

Bake for 15 to 20 minutes, or until the fish flakes easily with a fork. Remove from the oven and unwrap from the foil. Transfer to a plate and serve.

GINGER-LIME SALMON WITH ASPARAGUS

SERVES 1

1/3 cup low-sodium soy sauce

1/4 cup fresh lime juice

1 teaspoon minced fresh ginger

1/2 teaspoon chopped fresh thyme

2 garlic cloves, chopped

1 (6- to 8-ounce) salmon fillet

10 to 15 asparagus stalks, ends trimmed

In a small bowl, combine the soy sauce, lime juice, ginger, thyme, and garlic. Set the marinade aside.

Place the salmon in an oven-proof glass baking dish. Pour the marinade over the salmon and let it sit in the refrigerator, covered, for 60 minutes.

Preheat the broiler to medium. Remove the dish from the fridge and add the asparagus. Broil for 8 minutes. Halfway through, flip the salmon over, stir the asparagus, and continue to broil for another 4 minutes, or until the salmon is flaky and the asparagus are browning.

Remove from the oven, transfer to a plate, and serve.

GLUTEN-FREE VEGGIE PASTA

SERVES 1

2 handfuls of fresh spinach

1 cup sliced mushrooms

1 cup cherry tomatoes

1 garlic clove, minced

1 tablespoon olive oil

1/4 cup chopped fresh basil (or use frozen herbs)

6 ounces grilled chicken, precooked shrimp, or pan-seared scallops (optional)

¾ cup cooked brown rice pasta or quinoa pasta

2 tablespoons shaved Parmesan cheese

In a large pan over medium heat, sauté the spinach, mushrooms, tomatoes, and garlic in the oil until tender. Add the basil at the very end to preserve its flavor.

In a medium bowl, toss the vegetables, protein (if using), and pasta. Sprinkle with cheese and serve.

GRILLED HERBED CHICKEN WITH SPICY STRING BEANS

SERVES 1

FOR THE GRILLED HERBED CHICKEN

¼ cup fresh lemon juice

1 tablespoon chopped fresh parsley

1 tablespoon chopped fresh chives

1 teaspoon chopped fresh rosemary

1 garlic clove, minced

2 tablespoons olive oil

1 teaspoon salt

¼ teaspoon pepper

1 boneless skinless chicken breast

FOR THE SPICY STRING BEANS

12 ounces string beans

Zest of 1 lemon

1 tablespoon chopped parsley

2 tablespoons freshly grated Parmesan cheese

½ teaspoon red pepper flakes

¼ cup toasted and roughly chopped macadamia nuts

2 tablespoons olive oil

1 garlic clove, minced

1/2 teaspoon salt

To maked the grilled herbed chicken: In a small bowl, combine the lemon juice, parsley, chives, rosemary, garlic, oil, salt, and pepper. Whisk until well combined. Add the chicken breast and, using clean hands, toss the chicken in the marinade until well coated. Cover and refrigerate for a minimum of 15 minutes, or up to 2 to 3 hours.

Heat a grill or indoor grill pan to medium-high heat.

Remove the chicken from the refrigerator and cook it for 6 to 7 minutes on each side per inch of thickness. If the chicken breast is very thin, you may shorten the cooking time to 4 to 5 minutes per side.

Once the chicken is cooked, remove from the grill and transfer to a plate.

To make the spicy string beans: Bring a large pot of water to a boil. Add the beans and blanch for 3 minutes, until crisp yet tender. Drain the beans and immediately put them in a large bowl of ice water. Called "shocking," this process stops the cooking and sets the color. Let the beans sit in the ice water for at least 2 minutes.

In a small bowl, toss together the lemon zest, parsley, Parmesan, red pepper flakes, and nuts. Set aside.

When ready to serve, drain the beans and pat dry with a paper towel. Heat the olive oil in a large pan over medium-high heat. Add the beans to the pan and sauté for 2 minutes, or until heated through. Add the garlic and cook for another 30 to 60 seconds.

Remove from the heat, add the nut mixture, and toss well until all the beans are coated.

Sprinkle with salt and serve on the plate with the grilled chicken.

GRILLED PORK AND PEPPERS WITH
CREAMY SWEET POTATO MASH

SERVES 1

FOR THE GRILLED PORK

    5 to 6 ounces pork tenderloin

    1/2 teaspoon olive oil

    1/2 teaspoon salt

    1/2 teaspoon pepper

    1/2 teaspoon onion powder

    Vegetable oil cooking spray

FOR THE PEPPER

    1 bell pepper (red, yellow, or orange)

    1 teaspoon olive oil

    1/4 teaspoon salt

    1/4 teaspoon pepper

    1/4 teaspoon onion powder

FOR THE CREAMY SWEET POTATO MASH

    1 medium sweet potato

    2 tablespoons unsweetened coconut or almond milk

    1/4 teaspoon salt

    1/4 teaspoon pepper

To make the grilled pork: Heat a grill or indoor grill pan to medium-high heat. Lightly brush the pork with oil and sprinkle with salt, pepper, and onion powder evenly on both sides. Lightly spray the grill with the cooking spray, add the pork, and cook for 5 to 6 minutes on each side. Remove from the pan and let rest on a plate.

To make the pepper: Cut big wedges of the bell pepper off the core. In a small bowl, lightly toss the pepper wedges with oil, salt, pepper, and onion powder. If using a grill pan, use the same pan. Grill the pepper wedges on each side for 3 to 4 minutes, until they begin to soften and char. Transfer to the plate with the pork.

To make the creamy sweet potato mash: Peel the sweet potato and chop it into 2-inch cubes. Place the potato in a pot filled with cold water, just enough to cover the potato by 1 inch. Bring the water to a boil and cook for 10 to 12 minutes, until the potato is soft and can be pierced easily with a fork.

Once the potato is cooked, drain and then return the potato to the pot. Add the coconut milk, salt, and pepper. Use a potato masher or a fork to mash everything together. Transfer to the plate with the pork and pepper and serve.

KALE QUINOA CHOP

SERVES 1

1 (6- to 8-ounce) chicken breast, cooked and cubed
2 cups chopped fresh kale
2 cups chopped romaine lettuce
1/2 cup cooked quinoa
1/4 cup golden raisins
1/8 cup toasted sliced almonds
3 tablespoons lemon juice
1 tablespoon olive oil

In a small bowl, toss the chicken, kale, romaine, quinoa, raisins, and almonds. In a separate bowl, whisk the lemon juice and oil to make the dressing. Toss the salad with the dressing and serve.

LEMON PEPPER GRILLED STEAK SALAD

FOR LEMON PEPPER GRILLED STEAK

6 to 8 ounces sirloin steak

1 tablespoon olive oil

1/2 teaspoon salt

1/2 teaspoon lemon pepper

FOR THE SALAD

1/3 head romaine lettuce

1/2 cup halved cherry tomatoes

1/4 cup shaved Parmesan cheese

Balsamic vinegar, for drizzling

To make the lemon pepper grilled steak: Heat a grill or indoor grill pan to medium-high heat. Lightly brush the steak with oil. In a small bowl, combine the salt and lemon pepper and evenly sprinkle over both sides of the steak.

Cook the steak for 4 to 5 minutes on each side. Remove from the heat and let the steak sit for 5 to 10 minutes before slicing.

To make the salad: Place the lettuce on a plate. Top with the steak, followed by the tomatoes. Sprinkle the Parmesan over the salad and drizzle with the balsamic vinegar. Serve.

LETTUCE-WRAPPED TURKEY BURGER WITH BAKED SWEET POTATO

SERVES 1

FOR THE LETTUCE-WRAPPED TURKEY BURGER

1 turkey patty, store-bought or homemade (see Notes)

1/2 teaspoon salt

1/4 teaspoon pepper

1/2 teaspoon garlic powder

1/4 teaspoon paprika

Vegetable oil cooking spray

1 large leaf iceberg or romaine lettuce

FOR THE BAKED SWEET POTATO

1 medium sweet potato

Salt and pepper, to taste (optional)

To make the lettuce-wrapped turkey burger: Sprinkle the turkey patty evenly on both sides with salt, pepper, garlic powder, and paprika. Heat a nonstick skillet over medium-high heat. Lightly spray the skillet with the cooking spray and add the turkey patty. Cook for 5 to 7 minutes per inch of thickness on each side.

Remove from the pan and let rest for 3 to 5 minutes. Transfer to a plate and wrap in lettuce to finish.

To make the baked sweet potato: Preheat the oven to 400°F. Using a fork, prick some holes all over the sweet potato. Wrap in foil and bake for 45 to 55 minutes, until a knife is easily inserted into the center. Slice the potato open and sprinkle with salt and pepper (if using). (See Notes for microwave option.) Transfer to the plate with the burger and serve.

NOTES

To make a homemade turkey patty, you will need 5 ounces 93% lean ground turkey. In a bowl, use a fork to combine the meat and spices.

Use your hands to form the meat into a patty and cook according to the directions.

To cook a sweet potato in the microwave, simply prick some holes all over the sweet potato, wrap it in a wet paper towel, place in the microwave on a microwave safe-dish, and cook for 5 to 7 minutes, or until soft. DO NOT USE FOIL IN THE MICROWAVE!

MAMA WIDERSTROM'S GRILLED CAESAR SALAD WITH SKIRT STEAK

SERVES 1

FOR THE SKIRT STEAK

> 6 to 8 ounces skirt steak
>
> 1 to 2 tablespoons olive oil
>
> 1/2 teaspoon salt
>
> 1/2 teaspoon pepper
>
> 1/2 teaspoon garlic powder
>
> Vegetable oil cooking spray

FOR THE DRESSING

> 1 large egg
>
> 2 anchovy fillets
>
> 1 large garlic clove
>
> Pepper, to taste
>
> Juice of 1/2 lemon
>
> 2 tablespoons freshly grated Parmesan cheese
>
> 1/4 cup extra-virgin olive oil
>
> 1 teaspoon Dijon mustard, such as Grey Poupon
>
> 1 teaspoon Worcestershire sauce
>
> 2 or 3 dashes of hot sauce, such as Tabasco

FOR THE SALAD

> 1 head romaine lettuce
>
> 1 tablespoon olive oil
>
> Salt, to taste
>
> Pepper, to taste

To make the skirt steak: Brush the skirt steak with oil and sprinkle with salt, pepper, and garlic powder. Heat a large skillet over medium-high heat. Spray the skillet with the cooking spray and add the skirt steak. Cook for 3 to 5 minutes on each side. Remove from the pan and let rest for 5 to 10 minutes before slicing.

To make the dressing: Bring a saucepan of water to a boil. Add the egg and let cook for 45 seconds. Drain and set aside.

Add the anchovies, garlic, and pepper to the blender (see Note) and pulse until the garlic and anchovies are chopped and somewhat combined. Add the egg, lemon juice, and Parmesan and blend until well combined. Add the oil and blend until fully integrated and slightly thickened. Finally, add the Dijon mustard, Worcestershire sauce, and hot sauce and blend well.

Refrigerate for 10 to 15 minutes to allow flavors to blend.

To make the salad: While the dressing is in the fridge, prepare a charcoal or gas grill for direct grilling over medium heat. Take the head of romaine and quarter it, leaving the core intact. Place on a baking sheet, drizzle with olive oil, and season with salt. Toss gently. Place on the grill cut side down and grill until nicely marked (usually 1 to 2 minutes). Turn and mark the other side (again, 1 to 2 minutes).

Transfer the salad to a plate. Remove the dressing from the fridge and drizzle it over the salad. Add a few grinds of fresh pepper to taste. Place the slices of grilled skirt steak over the salad and serve.

NOTE
If you don't have a blender, use a fork to mash the anchovies, garlic, and pepper together before adding the other ingredients. Then simply use a whisk to combine the remaining ingredients.

ONE-POT CAULIFLOWER RICE PAELLA

SERVES 2

12 shrimp, peeled and deveined
1 teaspoon salt, plus a pinch
$1/2$ teaspoon turmeric
$1/2$ teaspoon smoked paprika
2 to 3 tablespoons olive oil

8 ounces cooked chicken sausage, sliced

1 small onion, chopped

1 red bell pepper, diced

1 orange bell pepper, diced

4 garlic cloves, minced

1 tablespoon tomato paste

4 cups Cauliflower Rice (recipe follows)

1/3 cup chicken stock or water

1 cup halved cherry tomatoes

1/2 cup frozen peas

Juice of 1 lemon (optional)

In a small bowl, toss the shrimp with 1/4 teaspoon of the salt, 1/4 teaspoon of the turmeric, 1/4 teaspoon of the paprika, and 1 tablespoon of the oil.

Heat a large pan or pot over medium heat. Add the shrimp and cook for 3 minutes on each side. Remove from the pan and set aside.

Add 1 tablespoon of the oil to the same pan and cook the chicken sausage for 5 to 7 minutes, until browned. Remove the sausage from the pan and set aside.

There may be enough oil still in the pan; if not, add the remaining 1 tablespoon oil and the onion, bell pepper, and a pinch of salt, and cook for 5 minutes. Add the garlic and cook for 1 more minute. Add the tomato paste and stir to coat.

Add the cauliflower rice and the remaining 3/4 teaspoon salt, 1/4 teaspoon turmeric, and 1/4 teaspoon paprika, and cook for 2 to 3 minutes, stirring occasionally.

Add the stock and cook until the liquid evaporates, 3 to 4 minutes.

Add the tomatoes and peas and heat through for a couple of minutes. Return the shrimp and sausage to the pan and stir to combine. Remove from the heat.

Transfer to a plate, drizzle the lemon juice (if using) over to finish, and serve.

CAULIFLOWER RICE

MAKES ABOUT 4 CUPS

1 pound cauliflower

Remove the leaves and stem from the cauliflower and discard. In a large bowl, grate the entire head of cauliflower until it resembles rice.

ONE-POT CHICKEN

SERVES 2

2 to 3 chicken breasts
3/4 tablespoon salt
1/2 teaspoon lemon pepper
1/4 teaspoon garlic powder
1/4 teaspoon onion powder
1/2 teaspoon paprika
1 tablespoon olive oil
1/3 cup rice wine vinegar
1/4 cup balsamic vinegar
2 tablespoons Dijon mustard
1 tablespoon honey
1 pint cherry tomatoes
Chopped fresh herbs, about 1/3 cup each of chives, parsley, and
  basil

Preheat the oven to 400°F.

Using paper towels, pat the chicken dry. In a small bowl, whisk together the salt, lemon pepper, garlic powder, onion powder, and paprika. Sprinkle the mixture evenly over the chicken on both sides. In a large pan, heat the oil over medium-high heat. Add the chicken and cook for 4 to 5 minutes on each side, until nicely browned. Add the rice wine vinegar to the pan. This will help to deglaze the pan. Cook for 1 to 2 minutes until most of the vinegar has cooked down. Remove from the heat and transfer the chicken to a baking dish.

In a small bowl, stir together the balsamic vinegar, Dijon mustard, and honey. Pour over the chicken, making sure the chicken is well coated. Cover the dish with foil and bake for 15 minutes. Remove the dish and add the tomatoes. Cover and bake for another 5 minutes, until the tomatoes are heated through and start to burst. Remove from the oven and discard the foil. Sprinkle with fresh herbs, transfer to a plate, and serve.

ONE-POT MEXICAN QUINOA

SERVES 2

2 tablespoons olive oil

1 onion, diced

2 boneless skinless chicken breasts, cubed (see Note)

2 garlic cloves, minced

$1/2$ teaspoon salt, plus more to taste

Black pepper, to taste

1 bell pepper (any color), diced small

1 cup black beans, rinsed and drained

1 ($14^1/2$-ounce) can diced tomatoes, not drained

1 teaspoon chili powder

$1/2$ teaspoon ground cumin

$1/2$ cup cooked quinoa

$1^1/2$ cups chicken stock (see Note)

Optional garnishes: diced avocado, chopped cilantro, and lime wedges

Juice of $1/2$ lime

In a large pan, heat the oil over medium-high heat. Add the onion and cook for 1 minute. Add the chicken, garlic, and a pinch of salt and pepper. Cook for 5 to 7 minutes until the chicken is no longer pink. Add the bell pepper, black beans, tomatoes, chili powder, cumin, the $1/2$ teaspoon salt, and black pepper to taste, and stir.

Add the quinoa and stock and stir to combine. Bring to a boil, then reduce the heat to low. Cover and simmer for 15 to 20 minutes. Remove from the heat, fluff with a fork, and serve with your desired garnishes. Add the lime juice to bring out all the flavors! Transfer to a plate and serve.

NOTE
You can easily make this dish vegetarian by leaving out the chicken and using vegetable stock instead of chicken stock.

OVEN-BAKED SALMON WITH ROASTED BRUSSELS SPROUTS AND ALMONDS

SERVES 1

FOR THE OVEN-BAKED SALMON
- 6 ounces salmon
- 1 teaspoon olive oil
- 1/4 teaspoon salt
- 1/2 teaspoon lemon pepper
- 1 lemon

FOR THE VEGGIES
- 1 cup halved Brussels sprouts
- 1 tablespoon olive oil
- 1/2 teaspoon salt
- 1/4 teaspoon lemon pepper
- 1/4 teaspoon garlic powder
- 2 teaspoons toasted slivered almonds
- 1 to 2 tablespoons crumbled goat cheese (optional)

Preheat the oven to 375°F.

To make the oven-baked salmon: Place the salmon in a baking dish. Brush the salmon with the oil and sprinkle evenly with the salt and lemon pepper. Cut two thin slices of lemon and place them on top of the salmon.

Bake for 20 to 25 minutes, until the fish is flaky. Remove from the oven, transfer to a plate, and squeeze the juice of the remaining lemon over the top to finish.

To make the veggies: Place the Brussels sprouts in a single layer on a sheet pan. Toss with oil, salt, lemon pepper, and garlic powder. Roast for 30 to 35 minutes, until slightly browned and tender. Stir the veggies halfway through the cooking time. Remove from the oven, toss in the almond slivers and goat cheese (if using), and transfer to the plate with the fish. Serve.

NOTES

Fish and veggies can cook in the oven at the same time.

Veggies can also be made ahead of time and stored in the fridge.

You can buy toasted almonds, or you can buy them raw and toast them in the oven yourself at 375°F. for 3 to 5 minutes. Watch them carefully! Or toast them in a dry pan for the same amount of time until golden brown.

PAN-SEARED SALMON WITH GARLICKY KALE

SERVES 1

1 (5-ounce) salmon fillet

1/2 teaspoon salt, plus more to taste

1/4 teaspoon pepper, plus more to taste

Vegetable oil cooking spray

1 tablespoon olive oil

2 cups chopped fresh kale

2 to 3 garlic cloves, minced

1/4 cup toasted pine nuts

Season the salmon evenly on both sides with the 1/2 teaspoon salt and the 1/4 teaspoon pepper. Spray a small skillet with the cooking spray. Place the salmon in the skillet and cook over medium heat for 5 to 6 minutes on both sides, until the salmon flakes easily with a fork. Set aside on a plate but keep warm.

In the same skillet, heat the oil over medium heat. Add the kale and garlic and cook for 3 to 5 minutes, stirring often, until the kale is tender. Add a pinch of salt and pepper and top with the pine nuts. Transfer to the plate with the salmon and serve.

PAN-SEARED SKIRT STEAK AND VEG

SERVES 1

FOR THE PAN-SEARED SKIRT STEAK

5 to 6 ounces skirt steak

1 to 2 tablespoons olive oil

1/2 teaspoon salt

1/2 teaspoon pepper

1/2 teaspoon garlic powder

Vegetable oil cooking spray

FOR THE BAKED SWEET POTATO

1 medium sweet potato

Salt and pepper, to taste (optional)

FOR THE ASPARAGUS

8 ounces asparagus stalks, ends trimmed

1 teaspoon olive oil

1/4 teaspoon salt

1/4 teaspoon pepper

1/4 teaspoon garlic powder

1 lemon

To make the pan-seared skirt steak: Brush the skirt steak with the oil and sprinkle with the salt, pepper, and garlic powder. Heat a large skillet over medium-high heat. Spray the skillet with the cooking spray and add the skirt steak. Cook for 3 to 5 minutes on each side. Remove from the pan and let rest on a plate for 5 to 10 minutes before serving.

To make the baked sweet potato: Preheat the oven to 400°F. Using a fork, prick some holes all over the sweet potato. Wrap in foil and bake for 45 to 55 minutes, until a knife is easily inserted into the center. Remove from the oven and discard the foil. Slice the potato open and sprinkle with the salt and pepper (if using). (See Note for microwave option.) Transfer to the plate with the steak.

To make the asparagus: Preheat the broiler. Place the asparagus on a sheet pan. Toss with the oil, salt, pepper, and garlic powder. Place the asparagus under the broiler for about 5 minutes, until lightly browned and tender-crisp. Remove from the broiler and drizzle with lemon juice over the top to finish. Transfer to the plate with the steak and potato and serve.

NOTE

To cook a sweet potato in the microwave, simply prick some holes all over the sweet potato, wrap it in a wet paper towel, place in the microwave on a microwave-safe dish, and cook for 5 to 7 minutes, or until soft. DO NOT USE FOIL IN THE MICROWAVE!

PROTEIN-STYLE TURKEY BURGER WITH CUBED SWEET POTATOES

SERVES 1

FOR THE PROTEIN-STYLE TURKEY BURGER

> 1 (5- to 6-ounce) turkey patty, store-bought or homemade (see Note)
>
> 1/2 teaspoon salt
>
> 1/4 teaspoon pepper
>
> 1/2 teaspoon garlic powder
>
> 1/4 teaspoon paprika
>
> Vegetable oil cooking spray
>
> 1 large butter lettuce leaf
>
> Optional garnishes: tomato, ketchup, mustard, and pickles

FOR THE SWEET POTATOES

1½ cups cubed sweet potato

1 tablespoon olive oil

½ teaspoon salt

½ teaspoon chili powder

To make the protein-style turkey burger: Sprinkle the turkey patty evenly on both sides with salt, pepper, garlic powder, and paprika. Heat a nonstick skillet over medium-high heat. Lightly spray the skillet with the cooking spray and add the turkey patty. Cook for 5 to 7 minutes per inch of thickness on each side.

Remove from the pan and let rest on a plate for 3 to 5 minutes before serving. Wrap the burger in the lettuce and top with your desired garnishes.

To make the sweet potatoes: Preheat the oven to 400°F. On a large baking sheet, toss the sweet potato cubes with the oil, salt, and chili powder. Bake for 20 to 25 minutes, until crispy brown on the outside and soft inside. Remove from the oven and transfer to the plate with the burger.

NOTE

To make a homemade turkey patty, you will need 5 ounces 93% lean ground turkey. In a bowl, use a fork to combine the meat and spices. Use your hands to form the meat into a patty and cook according to the directions.

ROASTED HALIBUT WITH VEGGIE MEDLEY

SERVES 1

1½ cups cauliflower florets

1½ cups chopped carrot

1½ cups broccoli florets

3 tablespoons olive oil, plus more for brushing

1 teaspoon salt, plus more to taste

½ teaspoon pepper, plus more to taste

1 (6-ounce) halibut fillet

Pinch of dried thyme

Juice of 1/2 lemon

Preheat the oven to 400°F.

Toss the cauliflower, carrot, and broccoli on a small sheet pan with the 3 tablespoons oil, the 1 teaspoon salt, and the 1/2 teaspoon pepper. Roast for 20 to 25 minutes, stirring halfway through the cooking time. Remove from the oven and transfer to a plate.

Place the halibut in a baking dish. (See Note.) Brush the fish with oil and sprinkle with salt, pepper, and thyme. Bake for 10 to 12 minutes. Remove from the oven and drizzle the lemon juice over to finish. Transfer to the plate with the veggies and serve.

NOTE

You can add the fish to the oven in the last 10 to 15 minutes of cooking time for the veggies so they're done at the same time.

SALMON BAKES

SERVES 1

Vegetable oil cooking spray

6 ounces salmon

1 bundle green onions (scallions), white and green parts, chopped

1/2 teaspoon salt

1/4 teaspoon pepper

Juice of 1 lemon

1 tablespoon extra-virgin olive oil

2 cups fresh baby kale

4 ounces cubed sweet potato

1 cup shaved Brussels sprouts

5 to 6 asparagus stalks, ends trimmed

Preheat the oven to 350°F. Lightly spray a glass baking dish with the cooking spray.

Chop up the salmon and mash it into a patty with the scallions, salt, pepper, lemon juice, and oil. Place the kale in the bottom of the prepared baking dish. Top with the salmon patty, sweet potato, Brussels sprouts, and asparagus. Bake for 15 to 18 minutes, or until the vegetables are tender and the salmon patty is cooked through to your preference. Remove from the over, transfer to a plate, and server.

SHRIMP PASTA

SERVES 1

Fresh minced garlic, to taste
Chopped fresh basil, to taste
Salt and black pepper, to taste
Red pepper flakes, to taste
1 tablespoon olive oil
8 asparagus stalks, ends trimmed, chopped into 1-inch pieces
6 ounces cooked shrimp
1 cup cooked brown rice pasta
2 cups fresh spinach
1/4 cup shaved Parmesan cheese

In a skillet over low heat, sauté the garlic, basil, salt, black pepper, and red pepper flakes in the oil. Add the asparagus and shrimp and cook for 3 to 5 minutes, or until the asparagus is bright green. Add the pasta and spinach. Fold together and cook until the spinach is gently wilted. Transfer to a plate, top with Parmesan, and serve.

SIMPLE STEAK FILET WITH MUSHROOM AND ASPARAGUS QUINOA

SERVES 1

1 (6-ounce) steak filet

1 tablespoon olive oil, plus more for brushing

Salt and pepper, to taste

Vegetable oil cooking spray

1/4 cup chopped onion

1/2 cup chopped mushrooms

6 asparagus stalks, ends trimmed, chopped

3/4 cup cooked quinoa

Heat a pan over medium-high heat. Brush the steak with the oil and sprinkle with the salt and pepper. Spray the pan with the cooking spray and add the steak. Cook for 5 to 6 minutes on each side. Remove from the pan and let rest on a plate while you put together the quinoa.

Use the same pan to cook your veggies. Add the 1 tablespoon oil, then add the onion, mushrooms, and asparagus to the pan with a sprinkle of salt and pepper. Cook for 7 to 10 minutes, until the veggies begin to soften. Toss with the cooked quinoa. Transfer to the plate with the steak and serve.

SKIRT STEAK AND ROASTED BRUSSELS SPROUTS

SERVES 1

5 to 6 ounces skirt steak

2 tablespoons olive oil, plus more for brushing

Salt and pepper, to taste

1/2 teaspoon garlic powder

Vegetable oil cooking spray

3 cups Brussels sprouts

3 garlic cloves, minced

Preheat the oven to 400°F.

Brush the skirt steak with the oil and sprinkle lightly with the salt, pepper, and garlic powder. Heat a large skillet over medium-high heat. Spray the skillet with the cooking spray and add the skirt steak. Cook for 3 to 5 minutes on each side. Remove from the pan and let rest for 5 to 10 minutes on a plate.

On a sheet pan, toss the Brussels sprouts and garlic with the 2 tablespoons oil and a large pinch of salt and pepper. Roast for 22 to 25 minutes, or until browned and tender, shuffling the vegetables at the halfway mark. Remove from the oven and transfer to the plate with the steak. Serve.

SLOW COOKER CHICKEN FAJITAS

SERVES 2

2 frozen chicken breasts
1 cup salsa, any type
Vegetable oil cooking spray
1 onion, chopped
1 green bell pepper, chopped
1 cup cooked brown rice, or butter lettuce leaves

SEASONINGS TO TASTE
Garlic powder
Onion powder
Salt
Pepper
Cumin
Chili powder
Oregano

Place the frozen chicken in a slow cooker and season as desired. Pour the salsa over the chicken. Cover and cook on low for 6 to 7 hours, or on high for 5 to 6 hours. Shred the chicken with a fork and return it to the slow cooker.

Spray a medium skillet with the cooking spray and add the onion and bell pepper. Sauté over high heat until the vegetables become slightly charred. Remove from the heat and set aside.

Serve the chicken mixture over the brown rice, or wrapped in butter lettuce leaves, on a plate alongside the sautéed veggies.

SLOW COOKER SHREDDED CHICKEN 1.0

SERVES 2

2 boneless skinless chicken breasts
12 ounces of your favorite salsa
1/2 packet taco seasoning

Place all the ingredients in a slow cooker. Cook on high for 4 hours. Shred the chicken, transfer to a plate, and serve.

SLOW COOKER SHREDDED CHICKEN 2.0 (OVER ROMAINE)

SERVES 2

FOR THE SALSA

1 (14-ounce) can fire-roasted tomatoes
1 cup halved cherry tomatoes
1/2 cup chopped red onion
1 jalapeño, seeded and chopped (add another one if you like it spicy)
2 garlic cloves, chopped
1/2 cup chopped fresh cilantro

1$\frac{1}{2}$ teaspoons salt

$\frac{1}{2}$ teaspoon pepper

Juice of 1 lime

Salt, to taste

1 pound boneless skinless chicken breasts (2 breasts)

1 teaspoon salt

$\frac{1}{4}$ teaspoon garlic powder

$\frac{1}{8}$ teaspoon oregano

$\frac{1}{8}$ teaspoon onion powder

$\frac{1}{8}$ teaspoon ground cumin

To make the salsa (see Note): Place all the ingredients in a food processor or blender and pulse until well blended. Transfer to a bowl.

To make the shredded chicken: Place the chicken in a slow cooker. Sprinkle the chicken with the salt, garlic powder, oregano, onion powder, and cumin. Add enough salsa to just cover the chicken and cook on high for 2 hours. In the last 30 minutes of cooking, remove the chicken, shred it, and return it to the slow cooker to finish cooking. Transfer to a plate and serve.

NOTE

You may have extra salsa left over that you can use to top the chicken, along with any of the following:

$\frac{1}{2}$ avocado, pitted, peeled, and diced, or $\frac{1}{4}$ cup shredded sharp Cheddar cheese

$\frac{1}{4}$ cup chopped red onion

$\frac{1}{4}$ cup corn kernels

Chopped fresh cilantro

SLOW COOKER SWEET POTATO CHILI

SERVES 3 TO 4

Vegetable oil cooking spray

1 pound sweet potatoes, peeled and cubed into $1/2$-inch dice

$1/2$ (15-ounce) can black beans, drained and rinsed

$1/2$ (15-ounce) can red kidney beans, drained and rinsed

1 cup chicken stock

1 (14-ounce) can diced tomatoes, undrained

$1/2$ onion, chopped

$1\frac{1}{2}$ teaspoons chili powder

3 garlic cloves, minced

$3/4$ teaspoon salt

$1/2$ teaspoon pepper

8 ounces 90% lean ground beef or 93% lean ground turkey (optional)

Lightly spray the slow cooker with the cooking spray. Place all the ingredients in the slow cooker and mix gently. Cook on high for 4 to 5 hours, or on low for 7 to 8 hours, until the sweet potatoes are soft, or until the meat is cooked through (if using).

NOTE
Leftovers are freezer friendly!

SLOW COOKER TURKEY MEATBALLS WITH BAKED SWEET POTATO "CHIPS"

SERVES 3 TO 4

FOR THE SLOW COOKER TURKEY MEATBALLS

$1\frac{1}{4}$ pounds ground turkey meat

$1/2$ small onion, minced

2 garlic cloves, minced

¹/₄ cup panko or regular bread crumbs, plus more as needed

1 large egg, lightly beaten

¹/₄ cup grated Parmesan cheese

1 teaspoon tomato paste

1 teaspoon salt

¹/₂ teaspoon pepper

1 teaspoon dried oregano

1 teaspoon dried basil

1 (13-ounce) jar marinara sauce

FOR THE SWEET POTATO "CHIPS" (SERVES 1)

Vegetable oil cooking spray

1 medium sweet potato, sliced as thin and evenly as possible

Olive oil, for brushing

Salt, to taste

Garlic powder, to taste

To make the slow cooker turkey meatballs: In a large bowl, combine the turkey, onion, garlic, panko, egg, Parmesan, tomato paste, salt, pepper, oregano, and basil. Mix using a fork until combined. Do not overmix. If the mixture seems too wet, add 1 tablespoon bread crumbs at a time until it's easy to handle and form into balls.

Pour a small amount of marinara sauce into the slow cooker—just enough to cover the bottom. As you form the meatballs, place them in the slow cooker. I make larger meatballs (slightly larger than a golf ball comes to about 12). Pour the rest of the sauce over the meatballs and cook on low for 6 to 6¹/₂ hours (see Note).

To make the baked sweet potato "chips": Preheat the oven to 400°F. Lightly spray a baking sheet with the cooking spray. Lay the sweet potato slices in one even layer on the baking sheet.

Brush the slices lightly with oil and lightly sprinkle evenly with salt and garlic powder. Flip the slices and repeat on the other side. Bake for 20 to 25 minutes, until the edges are browned and crisp. Remove from the oven and transfer to a plate.

Place the turkey meatballs on the plate with the sweet potatoes and serve.

NOTE
Leftover meatballs are freezer friendly!

SOY-HONEY CHICKEN WITH BROCCOLI

SERVES 2

1 tablespoon extra-virgin olive oil, plus more as needed
2 boneless skinless chicken breasts, cut into 1-inch pieces
Salt and pepper, to taste
1 teaspoon garlic powder
2 tablespoons low-sodium soy sauce
1 tablespoon honey
2 garlic cloves, minced
1 teaspoon cornstarch
3 cups broccoli florets
1 tablespoon sesame seeds

In a large pan, heat the 1 tablespoon oil over medium-high heat. Add the chicken and sprinkle with a large pinch of salt and pepper and the garlic powder. Cook the chicken for about 5 minutes, until it is no longer pink and begins to brown.

Meanwhile, in a small bowl, whisk together the soy sauce, honey, garlic, and cornstarch. Set aside.

Once the chicken is lightly browned, add the broccoli. Cook for 3 to 5 minutes, until the broccoli turns bright green and just begins to soften. If the mixture seems too dry, add a little more olive oil. Add the soy sauce mixture and cook for 1 minute until the sauce thickens. Sprinkle with the sesame seeds. Transfer to a plate and serve.

SPICY STUFFED PEPPERS

SERVES 3

3 medium bell peppers (any color)

2 tablespoons olive oil

1 small onion, chopped

1 1/2 teaspoons salt, plus more to taste

1/4 teaspoon black pepper, plus more to taste

1/2 cup shredded carrot

8 ounces cremini mushrooms, stems removed, chopped

1 pound 93% lean ground turkey

1 teaspoon garlic powder

1/4 teaspoon oregano

1/4 teaspoon smoked paprika

1/2 teaspoon red pepper flakes, plus more to taste

2 tablespoons tomato paste

1 (28-ounce) can crushed tomatoes

1/2 cup cooked brown rice

1 large handful of roughly chopped fresh spinach

2 tablespoons chopped fresh basil

Juice of 1/2 lemon

1/2 cup shredded mozzarella cheese (optional)

3/4 cup chicken stock

Preheat the oven to 400°F.

Prepare the bell peppers by cutting them in half through the stem and removing the core. Place in a large baking dish, cut side up, and set aside.

Heat the oil in a large pan over medium-high heat. Add the onion and a pinch of salt and black pepper, and cook for 5 to 7 minutes. Add the carrot and mushrooms and cook for another 2 to 3 minutes, or until the vegetables are tender.

Add the turkey, the 1 1/2 teaspoons salt, the 1/4 teaspoon black pepper, the garlic powder, oregano, paprika, and the 1/2 teaspoon red pepper flakes, and break up the meat while incorporating all the spices. Cook for 5 to 7 minutes, until the meat is no longer pink.

Add the tomato paste and stir to combine. Add the crushed tomatoes and let the mixture simmer over low heat for 10 to 12 minutes, stirring occasionally. Adjust the seasonings, adding more salt, black pepper, or red pepper flakes to taste. Add the rice, spinach, and basil and stir to combine. Remove from the heat and add the lemon juice.

Spoon the turkey-veggies mixture into the halved bell peppers until nice and full. Top each pepper with a little bit of cheese (if using). Pour the stock into the bottom of the baking dish and cover the dish lightly with foil. Bake for 20 to 25 minutes, until the peppers are just tender.

Remove from the oven and discard the foil. Transfer to a plate and serve.

SPRING GREENS SUPER SALAD

SERVES 1

3 large pinches of salt
1 cup short pasta (gluten-free/brown rice)
1/2 pound asparagus stalks, ends trimmed, cut into 2-inch pieces
1/2 cup frozen peas
3 cups mixed greens
1/4 cup sliced almonds
1 grilled chicken breast, cut into cubes (optional)

FOR THE DRESSING
1 tablespoon olive oil
1 tablespoon fresh lemon juice
1/4 teaspoon salt
Pinch of pepper

Bring a large pot of water to a boil. Once boiling, add the salt and pasta. Cook until done, according to the package directions. Once the pasta is cooked, remove it from the pot and set aside in a bowl (but keep the pasta water boiling; you will reuse it for the veggies). Another option is to pour the pasta into a colander with another pot beneath it to catch all the hot water.

Add the asparagus and peas to the pasta water and cook for 2 minutes. When the veggies are cooked, remove them from the water and place immediately into an ice bath. This will help stop the cooking and set the bright green color! Let sit for a few minutes, then drain.

In a large salad bowl, combine the pasta, asparagus, peas, greens, and almonds and set aside.

To make the dressing: In a small bowl, whisk together the oil, lemon juice, salt, and pepper.

Drizzle the dressing over the salad and toss to coat. Top with the chicken (if using) and serve.

STRAWBERRY SPINACH SALAD

SERVES 1

4 cups fresh spinach
3/4 cup sliced strawberries
6 to 8 ounces grilled chicken breast, sliced
1/3 cup feta cheese crumbles
1/4 cup diced red onion
Balsamic vinaigrette salad dressing

Place the spinach on a plate. Top with the strawberries, followed by the chicken, feta cheese, and onion. Drizzle with the salad dressing and serve.

TURKEY BAKE

SERVES 1

Vegetable oil cooking spray

4 ounces 93% lean ground turkey

2 tablespoons diced onion

1 large egg, beaten

1/2 teaspoon salt

1/4 teaspoon pepper

1/4 teaspoon ground cumin

1/4 teaspoon dried thyme

2 cups fresh baby kale

1 cup cubed summer squash

1 cup cubed zucchini

Preheat the oven to 400°F. Spray a glass baking dish with the cooking spray.

In a bowl, gently mix the turkey, onion, egg, salt, pepper, cumin, and thyme, then form it into a patty. Arrange the kale, squash, and zucchini in the prepared dish. Add the turkey patty on top. Bake for 18 to 22 minutes or until the vegetables are tender and the turkey patty is cooked through to your preference.

Remove from the oven, transfer to a plate, and serve.

TURKEY BURGER WITH CARAMELIZED ONION AND BAKED SWEET POTATO "CHIPS"

SERVES 1

1 (5- to 6-ounce) turkey patty, store-bought or homemade (see Note)

1/2 teaspoon salt

1/4 teaspoon pepper

1/2 teaspoon garlic powder

1/4 teaspoon paprika

Vegetable oil cooking spray

1 teaspoon olive oil

1/2 onion, chopped

FOR THE SWEET POTATO "CHIPS"

Vegetable oil cooking spray

1 medium sweet potato, sliced as thin and evenly as possible

Olive oil, for brushing

Salt, to taste

Garlic powder, to taste

Sprinkle the turkey patty evenly on both sides with the salt, pepper, garlic powder, and paprika. Heat a nonstick skillet over medium-high heat. Lightly spray the skillet with the cooking spray and add the turkey patty. Cook for 7 to 9 minutes per inch of thickness on each side.

Meanwhile, heat the oil in a pan over medium heat. Add the onion and cook for 15 to 20 minutes, until the onion is very soft and starts to caramelize.

Remove the burger from the pan and let rest for 3 to 5 minutes on a plate. Top with the onions to finish.

To make the baked sweet potato "chips": Preheat the oven to 400°F. Lightly spray a baking sheet with the cooking spray. Lay the sweet potato slices in one even layer on the baking sheet.

Brush the slices lightly with the olive oil and lightly sprinkle evenly with the salt and garlic powder. Flip the slices and repeat on the other side. Bake for 20 to 30 minutes, until the edges are browned and crisp.

Remove from the over, transfer to a plate with the burger, and serve.

NOTE

To make a homemade turkey patty, you will need 5 to 6 ounces ground turkey meat. In a bowl, use a fork to combine the meat and spices. Use your hands to form the meat into a patty and cook according to the directions.

TURKEY BURGER SAMMIE WITH CHOPPED KALE SALAD

SERVES 1

FOR THE TURKEY BURGER SAMMIE

1 (5- to 6-ounce) turkey patty, store-bought or homemade (see Notes)

1/2 teaspoon salt

1/4 teaspoon black pepper

1/2 teaspoon garlic powder

1/4 teaspoon paprika

Vegetable oil cooking spray

1 slice whole-grain bread, lightly toasted

FOR THE KALE SALAD

2 cups finely chopped fresh kale (see Notes)

2 tablespoons toasted slivered almonds

2 tablespoons dried cranberries

FOR THE HERBED VINAIGRETTE

1/4 yellow onion

1 garlic clove

3 tablespoons apple cider vinegar

2 tablespoons fresh lemon or lime juice

Large handful of fresh herbs (use mostly basil and parsley, and if you want, a little mint)

1/4 cup olive oil

1/4 teaspoon cayenne pepper

1/2 teaspoon salt

1/4 teaspoon black pepper

To make the turkey burger sammie: Sprinkle the turkey patty evenly on both sides with the salt, black pepper, garlic powder, and paprika. Heat a nonstick skillet over medium-high heat. Lightly spray the skillet with the cooking spray and add the turkey patty. Cook for 7 to 9 minutes per inch of thickness on each side.

Remove from the pan and let rest for 3 to 5 minutes. Place on top of the toasted bread on a plate.

To make the kale salad: In a large bowl, combine the kale, almonds, and cranberries. Set aside.

To make the herbed vinaigrette: Place the onion, garlic, vinegar, lemon juice, herbs, oil, cayenne pepper, salt, and black pepper in a blender and blend until smooth. Pour the dressing over the salad, just enough to coat (see Notes), and toss.

Transfer the salad to the plate with the burger and serve.

NOTES

To make a homemade turkey patty, you will need 5 to 6 ounces ground turkey meat. In a bowl, use a fork to combine the meat and spices. Use your hands to form the meat into a patty and cook according to the directions.

Feel free to replace some of the kale with chopped fresh spinach.

The dressing recipe will make more than you need for the salad. Store the rest in the fridge and use throughout the week for other salads, or to drizzle over chicken, fish, or steak.

TURKEY MEAT SAUCE PASTA

SERVES 1

1 tablespoon olive oil

2 tablespoons chopped onion

5 to 6 ounces ground turkey

2 garlic cloves, minced

$1/2$ teaspoon salt

$1/4$ teaspoon black pepper

$1/2$ teaspoon red pepper flakes

1 cup finely chopped cauliflower florets

$1/2$ cup shredded carrot

1 teaspoon tomato paste

1 cup marinara sauce

1 to 2 cups cooked brown rice pasta (Trader Joe's makes a great Brown Rice and Quinoa Fusilli)

Heat a large skillet over medium-high heat. Add the oil and onion and cook for 2 minutes. Add the turkey, garlic, salt, black pepper, and red pepper flakes and cook for 6 to 8 minutes, until browned. Remove the turkey from the pan and set aside.

Add the cauliflower and carrot to the pan. Cook for 3 to 5 minutes, then add the tomato paste and marinara sauce and stir to combine. Add the turkey back to the pan and simmer over low heat for another 5 minutes. Serve on a plate over the pasta.

VEGGIE BASIL PASTA

SERVES 1

1 tablespoon olive oil

4 cups fresh spinach

1/2 cup sliced mushrooms

1/2 cup halved cherry tomatoes

1 teaspoon minced garlic

Handful of fresh basil

1/2 cup cooked brown rice pasta

Shaved Parmesan cheese, for garnish

4 to 6 ounces cooked shrimp, grilled chicken, or cooked beef (optional)

In a skillet over medium heat, heat the oil. Add the spinach, mushrooms, tomatoes, and garlic and sauté for 4 to 7 minutes, until tender. Add the basil and cook until wilted. Remove from the heat. Place the pasta on a plate and top with veggies. Sprinkle the dish with the shaved Parmesan cheese and top with the shrimp, chicken, or beef (if using).

ZUCCHINI PESTO PASTA SAUTÉ

SERVES 1

6 ounces specified protein (organic soy/tofu and nondairy
protein acceptable)

Juice of 1/2 lemon

1 1/2 teaspoons extra-virgin olive oil

1 zucchini, peeled into long, pasta-like strips

1 cup chopped fresh kale

1 cup chopped asparagus stalks

1 cup chopped broccolini

1/4 cup chopped green onions (scallions), white and green parts

Salt and pepper, to taste

2 tablespoons pesto

In a large pan over medium heat, sauté the protein with the lemon
juice and oil until browned on both sides and cooked throughout. Remove from the heat and set aside.

In a separate pan over medium heat, combine the zucchini, kale,
asparagus, broccolini, and onions. Add a few tablespoons of water,
season with salt and pepper, and cover. Cook for 4 to 7 minutes, until
the vegetables are bright green and still a bit crunchy.

Add the pesto and coat all the veggies with it. Add the protein and
heat thoroughly.

Remove from the heat. Mix well, transfer to a plate, and serve.

PART 3

MOVEMENT IS MEDICINE

CHAPTER 11

JOIN THE MOVEMENT

Your body is designed to move—so move it must! When asked about how to start a workout program, most people are surprised by the simplicity of my answer:

MOVE MORE, PERIOD

Take a moment to pause, and remove any preexisting fears relating to your perception of movement. Part of this chapter is about reframing your mind-set about your workouts, seeing them as an asset and *not* as an opportunity to fail. You will come to realize that bringing more movement into your life can be as simple as parking at the back of the lot at the mall or grocery store and walking to the door, or as intense as full-fledged weekly interval workouts with weight training.

One of my key mantras that I want you to adopt for yourself is "movement is medicine"—powerful preventative stuff that keeps your arteries clear, your body young, and your muscles strong; it also relieves stress and has even more benefits for our physical, mental, and emotional well-being. The changes and adaptations the body makes as a result of regular exercise are nothing short of amazing. Exercise ignites the body's immune system, improves mental function, boosts energy, burns body fat, and reduces the risk for chronic diseases such as heart disease, cancer, and diabetes.

New research on fitness says your genes, including anticancer genes, get fired up with exercise, and certain neurons in the brain light up, so your mood is elevated while fueling your workout from an emotional standpoint. Moving your body will help improve the meal choices you make and your ability to rest after a workout and will even create a more positive attitude. The more you move, the healthier you're going to be. Are we clear?

Keep this concept of *movement is medicine* tucked in your pocket because it will empower you and inspire you to move consistently. Physically, mentally, and emotionally, you'll feel more buoyant and free when you let yourself move more. And remember, movement transforms your mental health as much as it does your physical well-being.

Eventually, you'll get to a place in which exercise and physical activity become second nature, and when you don't move, you won't feel like yourself. Exercise will have a positive ripple on your entire life.

Making the shift toward an active lifestyle will be an epic turning point in your life. Once it takes place, you'll find yourself looking at the gym and even a group class differently. You'll walk toward it with a sense of pride, joy, and accomplishment, especially considering how you used to dislike exercise just months ago. Just as empowering will be looking at your days ahead with the anticipation of how much further you will be able to evolve and grow.

EXERCISE AND YOUR PERSONALITY

To help you get started and stay committed, consider your personality when deciding what exercise approach may be best for you. For some people, the idea of going for a walk or run by themselves is perfection. They feel that the alone time allows them to think, and they enjoy exercising at a time of their choosing. Others can't imagine anything more boring and isolating than working out alone and would prefer to be around other people, dancing or taking a spin class with killer music and club lights.

If your workout is not in line with who you are and what you enjoy, then you inherently won't want to stick to it. You'll be more likely to reject exercise without really knowing why. Thus, you need to be mindful of your personality, what setting you thrive in, and what you're willing to do for workout success. Laying out a plan of attack that suits you may be the difference between those who stick to exercise and those who wish they could.

Take a look at the following sections. Because my focus is about you *moving more*, I don't get super specific about what each personality type should do in the form of types of exercises. I do, however, include some clear personality-fitted guidelines to help you optimize your training success and home in on how you like to exercise.

In the final section of this chapter, I introduce you to my Jen Bod Workouts. They are a series of quick, effective routines that share the same workout template but work for any body, any personality type—anywhere. These are a great way to get your body on the move. I've also included a variety of movements and equipment to keep you engaged. These are excellent workouts to fall back on when you're tight on time. You can do them at home or at the gym.

But first, let's start with some general exercise advice matched to your personality.

> **JEN JUJU: Do Your Thang**
> *We spend a lot of time worrying about what other people are doing, and when they're doing it, and ultimately look to their success in order to define our own. However, through all the looking out we forget to look within to honor our own desires, energy, and timing. People always talk about the best time to train: the morning, the evening, what time burns the most calories, and so on. But if you're not a morning person, don't set yourself up for failure by committing to morning sessions—you'll only feel guilty when you hit snooze and skip your workout. The best time of day to sweat is the time that you'll actually do it!*

THE ORGANIZED DOER

You know how important exercise is to your well-being, and once you make up your mind to get active, you're all in. A structured program and a set schedule work best for you. A hard worker and diligent, you tend to be systematic in your workouts. You love details and aren't afraid of devoting long hours to training.

You're highly motivated by results, so keeping track of your progress is vital, whether it is number of reps, amount of weight, or duration or frequency of exercise. Organized Doers love to download their workout results in order to benchmark progress later. Therefore, you must track your improvements so you can see the positive changes you're making—no matter how big or small.

When working with Organized Doers, I advise them to set weekly goals that are appropriate for their fitness level. Because your expectations are often very high, talk with a fitness professional about your program and see if your goals are realistic. Perhaps have a workout buddy that you set goals with each week. It's important that you see clear signs of progress, such as having to buy a smaller size, because for you there is no greater reward. The key is to be realistic with your approach but appreciate the goals you set for yourself. With realistic benchmarks and a practical approach, you will quickly see your goals become reality.

Training-wise, it's best if your workout days don't waver. For example, set up your schedule so that you train every Monday, Wednesday, and Friday. If you're already a fitness buff, a Monday, Tuesday, Thursday, Friday, and Saturday training scheme works well.

If you're new to working out or haven't exercised in a while, I want you to do some homework. Test out a few gyms, workout techniques, classes, instructors, and so forth, to gain a sense of where, to what, and to whom you feel the most connected. Your comfort and trust in the effectiveness of the workout and/or trainer is everything when it comes to your level of commitment, but once you pick it, you're all in!

For Organized Doers, class settings and independent training systems are both effective. Brain-training activities are great for your personality type, too: boxing; Pilates; short, intense circuit training; and classes in which your in-room stats are being tracked and showcased. All of these approaches activate your mind in a way in which it's so busy being in the room that your daily worries are left at the door, and the workout acts not just as a calorie burner but also as a meditation.

THE SWINGER

Exercising is as much a social event for you as it is sweating. You look forward to the social interaction of going to the gym or exercise class sometimes more than the actual activity itself. If you try to work out on your own, it's unlikely that it will stick. You like accountability and camaraderie; it's what motivates you and excites you.

In fact, Swingers thrive on accountability. For you, meeting up with others or befriending your trainer, instructor, or class members is often a motivating factor behind keeping exercise consistent. It wouldn't surprise me to see you get a group of friends together and hire a trainer to teach a group class. If you're not interested in joining a gym, you'd do well in a walking or running group. However, your personality type can cut into the quality of your exercise program. If you spend too much time talking without enough action, your exercise efforts may be diminished.

Often, you're gung-ho to the point of excess, getting overly consumed with a workout in the beginning and then ultimately getting bored with it. Your all-in mentality switches to "good enough"; even then motivation wanes, and you're back to where you started. Your response: "Another workout that didn't work." But before long, you dive into the next exercise trend that comes along.

Still, you very much want to succeed but sometimes feel stuck and don't know how. Fear of failure often overshadows your total commitment to any sort of plan—which explains your tendency to move around from one activity to the next. This action undermines success because plans are never given the full opportunity to unfold.

Remember that Swingers don't thrive independently. You need a point person and/or a system for accountability so you don't fall short of daily and weekly commitments. Is it a personal trainer? A training app? Could it be a CrossFit studio that's heavily community based? An authentic belonging and relationship to your training preferences could be huge for you.

In Week 1, I'd like you to do the following benchmark to test yourself physically:

Test your 400-meter time and on a separate day test a full mile time, completing each as quickly as you can. I'd also like you to test your maximum number of sit-ups in 2 minutes. I'll have you retest all three at two-week increments so you can experience the success that you've been working for. You'll develop pride and confidence in the success that you'll see and *share* with your new community—all of which is enough to keep you going.

Check not only pounds and inches lost, but progress points such as enjoyment/continued interest. If you're below 60 to 65 percent of feeling engaged, move on! This doesn't mean you won't revisit this workout system, but for now we need to shelve it. Be creative and try something new. Add variety to keep exercise fun, maintain realistic expectations, and develop a new plan to achieve your goals. Don't always do the same workouts in the same order at the same time with the same weights, for example. Every workout should be a little bit different.

THE REBEL

When it comes to working out, most of the time you're actually quite motivated, but it's just a matter of logistically making it happen and giving it a place in your schedule. That means having packed a whole workout outfit but not forgetting to bring gym shoes or even making it all the way to a class but not being there at the correct time or day!

Most days, you live life hour by hour, so some days you may go to the gym, and some days you may not. You're so open-minded that if a window of time frees up and your gym bag is in the car, you'll hit up a workout without hesitation. But let's be honest, if you had to choose between happy hour and a workout, you'd head to the pub for quality friend time.

When you do hit the gym, you crank. You enjoy circuits and weights, all the way to a moving cycling session with good music and great messaging. You do best when you keep your commitment to exercise short and sweet—*and* in the morning. Logging your sweat session earlier in the day is critical for you because as the day goes on, training gets pushed farther and farther out of the priority position.

Your exercise schedule is so random that you neglect to set any tangible goals. It's thus been difficult for you to achieve a desirable level of fitness and/or weight loss in the process. I will say, however, out of any personality, you celebrate overall health, mental wellness, and a positive body image better than anyone.

Your success lies in reducing chaos through providing accessible patterns and habits that do not get in the way of your spontaneity.

I am establishing weekly minimums for the gym but without outlining specific days off or days on in that training schedule. Therefore, you will have "zero days off" because knowing you as well as I do, they will naturally occur. That being said, you cannot go beyond three days without a workout. So if things get a little chaotic and a naturally occurring day off turns into two days off, you cannot head to bed on day three without having to sweat it out sometime that day. Make sense? This means on any given week, you will never train less than two days. Within this, I will hold you to the following baseline expectations, allowing you to maintain a degree of freedom while still effectively living and losing:

- Workouts will be no less than forty-five minutes.
- Within each workout you must achieve elevated heart rate over time, forcing you to break a sweat (intervals included).
- You must eat directly after your workout (two servings of protein + one serving of carbohydrate + one serving of water).

Working with so many Rebel personalities, I've found that you all are up for and enjoy most everything. The key is sticking to the movement systems that have the greatest positive effect on your weight loss. For instance, if you find you're dropping weight faster going to a cycling class versus a boot camp class, but you enjoy both, you can still do boot camp—but prioritize those cycling classes in your plan.

If you're struggling to get the ball rolling, *get outside*. For your personality, the fresh air and freedom of space will innately inspire you and bring more pleasure to the experience—both of which will help get you over that initial movement hump.

Ultimately, you'll experience positive reinforcement from any form of progress, big or small: in your energy level, the way you look in the mirror, the way you feel, the mastery of a gym skill, or simply meeting your weekly minimum for the gym.

THE EVERYDAY HERO

Because you often tend to your own needs last, fitting in exercise can be a challenge. Unlike other personality types, you know exactly how to be successful in your fitness journey and have experienced it multiple times. Deep down, you know that a healthy body is an active body, and being healthy bolsters your ability to care for others. So when you fall short, you feel ashamed and put yourself down for not being consistent. That's the interior you, whereas the exterior you puts on a default front of "I'm fine."

You want people to see you as having it all together, all the time. Supportive, loyal, dependable, and a great motivator, you ironically are so good at being there for others in the way you sorely need support yourself. Perhaps that's why you're so good at it—because you need people to motivate you to exercise and know exactly what you need to hear to get you motivated, so you apply that intel with others.

When it comes to training, here is a weekly workbook of my expectations: Any on-the-fly workout will not be completed, so beginning your week I need you to schedule in your workouts just as you would a doctor's appointment or meeting a buddy for lunch. When you do, pad that time fifteen minutes on the front and back ends because you'll need the transition time in place in order for you to really be in your session for the forty-five to sixty minutes. Initially, I recommend that you have somebody at ground zero, such as a personal trainer for one to two sessions a week, to keep you accountable and build momentum. The reality of an Everyday Hero is that you would bail on time for yourself (aka your workout), but you *would never* bail on a person. That being said, a trainer will not only help you lock in those baseline sessions but also help you execute your training plans for the entire week.

Whether you are training in a private or group setting, focus on full workouts whenever you can, using a variety of movement systems, from moving your body weight to moving iron. Physically and mentally, you'll rise to the challenge while using your time very effectively.

I've seen the Everyday Hero gravitate toward the following types of workouts, especially in the beginning of their fitness journey:

Personal training
Boot camp/interval training classes (treadmill plus weights)
CrossFit
Pilates

Whether you work out in classes or independently, you'll be consistent because you know someone is counting on you to do it. If month one is about starting the engine, month two is about shifting it into a higher gear. You are so adaptable that you really only *need* one month to set yourself in motion. After that, you've got the capability to soar. Your metabolism will be supercharged, your workout stamina will be through the roof, and your sense of self will be powerfully elevated. All this translates to results you'll see in the mirror—and you'll love the empowered feeling of what you've accomplished.

THE NEVER-EVER

You've never really taken the time to identify what kind of exercise you prefer, but you inherently know how critical movement is for you. It's great therapy for you because you manifest your stress physically. Moving your body forces you to experience emotional breakthroughs that you otherwise would not have faced. This creates an opportunity for you to move through the energy that was getting you stuck and allows you to leave it behind. Bottom line, what you do in the gym translates far beyond its walls, if only you could get yourself there.

When I meet Never-Evers who don't want to exercise or have begun trying and are ready to quit, I confront them with some hardcore facts: a sedentary lifestyle will eventually catch up with you in many forms. For example, you could become obese—which can lead to depression, not wanting to go out of the house, or embarrassment when having to squeeze into an airplane seat. It can also lead to chronic back problems, in which you might not be able to pick up your kids or grandkids. Exercise prevents osteoporosis, which weakens bones. Lack of exercise can also lead to stiff, painful joints, blood sugar problems, a deconditioned heart, high blood pressure, and more. Most of these conditions can severely limit your ability to enjoy your life—and sadly but truthfully, even cut it short.

Consider: A study published in the esteemed medical journal *Annals of Internal Medicine* pointed to the fact that being overweight in our twenties, thirties, and forties can make part of our sixties, seventies, or eighties disappear. Dutch scientists reported that people who are overweight at forty are likely to die three years sooner than other forty-somethings who are thin. Further, obese forty-year-olds (more than 20 percent over healthy body weight) risked losing up to six to seven years of their lives. Getting rid of those pounds later in life may not completely reverse the danger, either. So even if you shed weight at an older age, you may still carry a higher risk of dying early.

I know you don't want that, and neither do your loved ones.

I hope that big-picture proof and scary statistics like these are enough to get you off the couch and into the gym. I've often recommended that Never-Evers get into the fitness groove gently—by wearing a pedometer that counts daily steps or taking the stairs versus the elevator. It doesn't seem like much initially, but once movement begins to feel accessible for you, you let go of that defeatist way of thinking and begin to live with a conquerable mind-set.

Picture an old coal train ... slow to start, perhaps, but once it gains momentum, nothing can compare to its strength, speed, and sheer power. Your workouts will shift from gentle walks after lunch to empowering activities that are interactive and easy to master. In this progression for you, I suggest boxing, yoga, and interval weight training. This can and will be you. It's going to take willpower to get your wheels to begin to move, but once you do, you will fight to protect the life you are building.

There is hope. Whether it's the feeling of accomplishment after a workout, the joy of a jog in the sunshine, or the self-control found in *not* finishing off that box of cookies, pay attention to the positive feelings that come with making healthy choices. Then use the power of that good choice as a motivator for more good. You will discover that you enjoy the challenges of eating well and staying active, and once you arrive here there's no way you'll go back to the "un-you" . . . unfit, unfulfilled, unhappy. You can't; it's simply not who you are anymore.

I suggest that you keep your workouts short and to the point (which is why you will love my Jen Bod Workouts). I'd like to see you do your workouts at home for now. Never-Evers who jump right into workouts focus only on obstacles and eventually find them too daunting.

Working out at home will be more convenient for you: no drive time, no need to put on makeup or fix your hair or find some cute gym outfit to wear. There's no pressure or self-consciousness when you train in the comfort of your own space, especially if you're not yet comfortable with the way you look.

JEN JUJU: Progress, Not Perfection

If someone said to you, "Run a mile," you might respond, "OMG, I haven't run a mile since I was ten years old in PE class." You feel fear, doubt, and even a degree of shame for being so out of touch with what is seemingly so easy for so many people.

Nonetheless, you want to run a mile. The best way to achieve that goal is to take small, progressive steps toward it. So you start by walking half a mile. Gradually, you start jogging half a mile. Then you run that half mile. After two months of training like this, you run a full mile. Now you have an accomplishment. Now you've gotten confident. Now you're tied to your success. If you say, "I want to be better. I want that measurable progress," when you see it, there's something empowering about achieving it because you lived and breathed every step of it. Now instead of carrying doubt, you carry pride and the willingness to step out of your comfort zone and accept a new challenge.

CHAPTER 12

JEN BOD WORKOUTS

No matter what your personality type is, I want you to move like an athlete. This is a baseline principle in the way I train my clients because it creates strong bodies with ideal contouring of the muscle, while also working muscle fibers in a way that achieves the highest calorie burn.

Let me elaborate a bit. There are three main types of muscle fibers in your body: fast-, slow-, and intermediate-twitch fibers. In the resistance programming I will provide, you will hit a combination of all three, but the plyometric components of the workouts will primarily recruit fast-twitch fibers, which happen to be the fibers that yield the greatest calorie burn. I've done this to accelerate your results and optimize your ability to get leaner, with more muscle definition—faster.

In my workouts, these concepts will be executed through a time-on-tension focus of resistance training, while incorporating movement patterns and explosive work sets that keep your body moving and your heart rate elevated.

The resistance training will include using your own body weight, resistance bands, and multiple forms of weights to achieve your body-shaping goals. It is designed to give you an invigorated muscle challenge and an effective way to firm up soft muscles.

One of my favorite aspects of resistance training is that when the workout comes to an end, your body doesn't stop burning calories. You actually continue burning calories for four, six, even eight hours afterward because the muscle tissue in your body is repairing and healing. So instead of just doing cardio, where once the action stops, the benefit stops, you will have the extended benefit of continued calorie burn well beyond the walls of the gym. This is the power of working and building muscle!

It's a little scary to consider, but research studies suggest that muscle strength and the tissue itself begin to fade when we enter our midthirties. In fact, fitness professionals estimate that one third to one half pound of muscle mass is lost per year, *every* year. That is what you can expect to lose if you stay inactive and don't introduce resistance training into your sweat sessions. Now some good news: strengthening your body significantly slows down the rate of muscle loss and, in many cases, stops it for years! Resistance training is the component you cannot afford to ignore any longer because when it comes to short- *and* long-term weight loss, plain cardio just won't cut it.

In this chapter you'll find instructions on how to perform a variety of fat-burning, muscle-developing exercises. I've folded them into eight 16-minute workouts so you will have a lot to choose from here to help keep you moving, and you'll never get bored. Best of all, since each workout is over in just 16 minutes and can be done at home, it is easy to squeeze into your day.

There's no excuse not to exercise anymore. Ready or not, here we go.

EXERCISE INSTRUCTIONS

BODYWEIGHT-ONLY EXERCISES

A-1: Reverse Lunges

Stand tall with your feet together and your hands behind your head. Step backward with one leg into a lunge position. As you step backward, lower your center of mass while keeping your back straight, chest open, and shoulders back. The goal is to have your rear knee about 1 inch off the ground and to keep your front knee completely vertical. Squeeze your buttocks while opening up the front of your hip (aka hip flexor).

From this position, transition back into the starting position by putting the pressure on your front foot and engaging your glute on that same leg to bring your back leg up to the starting position. Replicate the movement on the other side to complete one rep.

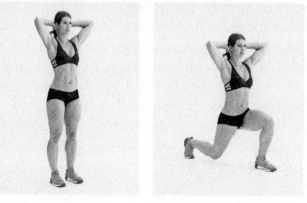

A-2: Mountain Climbers

Start in the push-up plank position, with your legs extended behind you, arms and body straight, with your hands directly below your shoulders. Bend your left leg and bring your knee up toward your left arm as far as you can. Reverse your movement and repeat with your right leg and right arm to complete one rep. Pick up the pace once you feel comfortable with the movement.

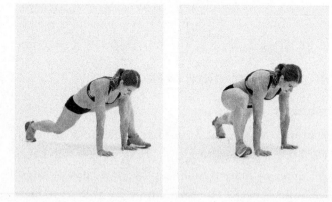

B-1: Plank Hold

Start in the push-up plank position, with your legs extended behind you, elbows slightly bent, hands directly below your shoulders, your core engaged, and your spine neutral. Be careful not to let your hips sink. Hold the plank for 60 seconds. As you improve, gradually increase the amount of time.

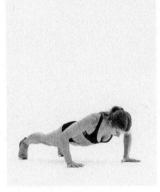

B-2: Push-ups (Full Range)

Begin in your plank position and lower your body to the ground. Slowly lower your chest to the floor by bending your elbows. Don't sag at the waist or arch your buttocks. Hold the down position for one count, then return to the starting position by extending your arms. If you're a beginner, you may also perform this exercise from a kneeling-start position.

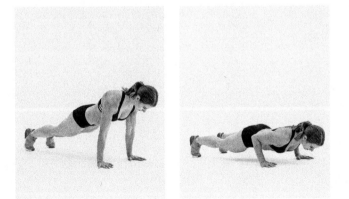

C-1: Alternating Side Squats

Stand with your feet placed far beyond your shoulder width. Step your right foot out to the side and squat down, leaning in toward your hip. Keep your hips back and over your heels while reaching your arms out in front of you for balance. Push off with your right foot back to center and repeat on the left side for one rep.

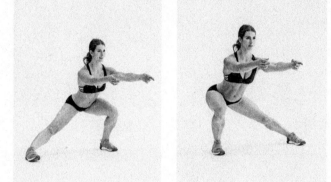

C-2: Burpees

Stand tall with your feet shoulder width apart. Bend down into a squat and put your hands on the ground. Pop your legs out behind you into a plank, and do a push-up. Hop your feet back to a standing position, finishing off with a little hop. Immediately begin the next burpee.

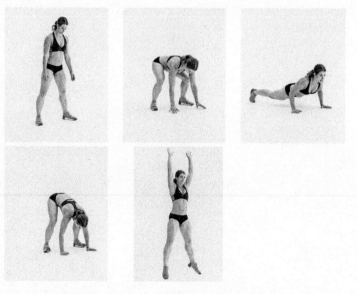

THE 16-MINUTE BODYWEIGHT-ONLY ROUTINE

To complete the routine, perform Sequences A, B, and C consecutively.

SEQUENCE A

Complete three rounds of the following; try to increase the number of reps each cycle:

A-1: Reverse Lunges: Do as many reps as you can in 30 seconds.

A-2: Mountain Climbers: Do as many reps as you can in 30 seconds.
Rest for 30 seconds.

Immediately following the third round, complete cardio-burst options for 90 seconds: running or jogging or marching in place; side shuffles; jumping jacks; or jump rope.

SEQUENCE B

Complete three rounds of the following; try to increase the number of reps each cycle:

B-1: Plank Hold: Hold for 30 seconds.

B-2: Push-ups (Full Range): Do as many reps as you can in 30 seconds.
Rest for 30 seconds.

Immediately following the third round, complete cardio-burst options for 90 seconds: running or jogging or marching in place; side shuffles; jumping jacks; or jump rope.

Complete three rounds of the following; try to increase the number of reps each cycle:

> **C-1: Alternating Side Squats:** Do as many reps as you can in 30 seconds.

> **C-2: Burpees:** Do as many reps as you can in 30 seconds.
> *Rest for 30 seconds.*

Immediately following the third round, complete cardio-burst options for 90 seconds: running or jogging or marching in place; side shuffles; jumping jacks; or jump rope.

JEN JUJU: Dial In to Your Workout Frame of Mind

Sometimes we lose momentum and motivation in our training, which raises the question: how do we get it back? Before I answer that, let me ask you: how did you lose that momentum in the first place? In my experience, it all comes from where we source our workouts. If you're exercising solely to lose weight, for an external experience, I'm here to warn you that your momentum isn't going to last. Your reasons for movement and exercising need to come from something deeper within you: I want to build the power of my promises to myself. I want to be vibrant and confident when I communicate. I want to be an energetic parent. I simply want to feel great about myself.

True confession: There are times when I just don't feel like working out, so I phone a friend to meet me for a workout. I would never stand my friend up. There's power in saying, "I said I would go, so I'm going." And frankly, my gym community is made up of people I love to be around.

For me, exercising is more than weight loss. I like to move because I feel better. I'm more alert in my day. I'm happier in my life. Those feelings are how I stay in a positive frame of mind. If you make exercising about the work, it will feel like work. If you make it about the experience, it will change your life.

RESISTANCE BAND EXERCISES

A-1: Standing Piston Press

Stand tall with your left foot forward. Place the center of the band under the arch of your left foot. Hold the handles of the band just above shoulder height in press position with your elbows bent. Press upward with one arm, then lower. Simultaneously press up with the other arm. Your arms should be pressing up and down, in alternating fashion, like a piston.

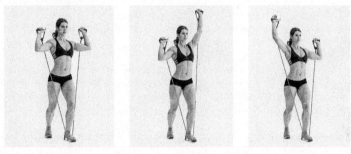

A-2: Bent-Over Row

Begin with your feet hip width apart. Place the band under the arches of both feet and grasp the handles in each hand. Cross the band, making an X with the handles. Bend forward at your waist, while keeping a straight back and engaging your core. Slowly and consistently, row the handles toward your chest, bringing your elbows up toward the ceiling and squeezing your shoulder blades together. Slowly return to the starting position to complete one rep.

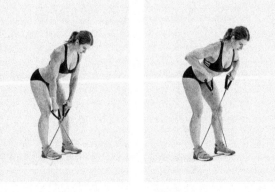

B-1: Full-Range Lateral Curls

Stand tall with your feet about hip width apart. Place the band under both feet and grasp the handles in each hand. Fully extend your arms out to each side, with your chest and shoulders fully open.

With your palms facing outward, grip the handle tightly. Flex your elbows and curl upward toward your head, until you can't curl any farther. Return your arms to the fully extended position to complete one rep.

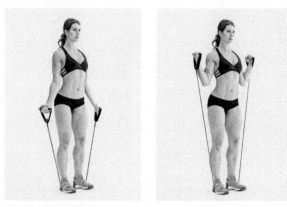

B-2: Door Hinges

Stand tall with your feet about hip width apart. Place the band under both feet and grasp the handles in each hand. Hold your elbows at 90 degrees with your palms facing up.

Continue holding your elbow at 90 degrees, but bring your arms together in front of you, just like a door opens and closes on its hinge, to complete one rep.

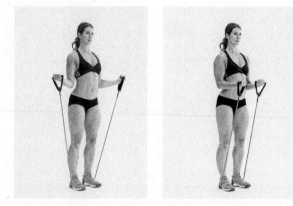

C-1: Side Steps (4s)

Stand tall with your feet shoulder width apart and place the band under your feet. Grasp the handles in each hand, with your palms facing upward in the 90-degree elbow position.

Lower your hips into a high-squat position. Take four large steps laterally, then take four more steps back to the starting position to complete one rep. Keep repeating this back-and-forth movement, never breaking the high-squat position or allowing your arms to release. Take about one second per step.

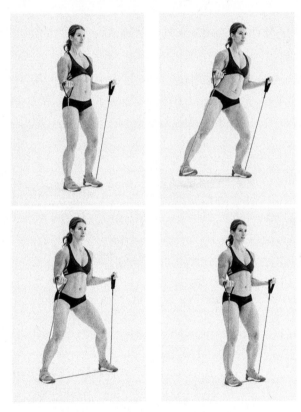

C-2: Advanced Side Steps (8s)

Stand tall with your feet shoulder width apart and place the band under your feet. Grasp the handles in each hand, with your palms facing upward in the 90-degree elbow position.

Lower your hips into a high-squat position. Take eight half steps moving laterally to one side, then take eight more half steps back to the starting position to complete one rep. Keep repeating this back-and-forth movement, never breaking the high-squat position or allowing your arms to release. Do these steps double-time.

THE 16-MINUTE RESISTANCE BAND ROUTINE

To complete the routine, perform Sequences A, B, and C consecutively.

SEQUENCE A

Complete three rounds of the following; try to increase the number of reps each cycle:

> **A-1: Standing Piston Press:** Do as many reps as you can in 30 seconds.

> **A-2: Bent-Over Row:** Do as many reps as you can in 30 seconds. *Rest for 30 seconds.*

Immediately following the third round, complete cardio-burst options for 90 seconds: running or jogging or marching in place; side shuffles; jumping jacks; or jump rope.

SEQUENCE B

Complete three rounds of the following; try to increase the number of reps each cycle:

> **B-1: Full-Range Lateral Curls:** Do as many reps as you can in 30 seconds.

> **B-2: Door Hinges:** Do as many reps as you can in 30 seconds. *Rest for 30 seconds.*

Immediately following the third round, complete cardio-burst options for 90 seconds: running or jogging or marching in place; side shuffles; jumping jacks; or jump rope.

SEQUENCE C

Complete three rounds of the following; try to increase the number of reps each cycle:

C-1: Side Steps (4s): Do as many reps as you can in 30 seconds.

C-2: Advanced Side Steps (8s): Do as many reps as you can in 30 seconds.

Rest for 30 seconds.

Immediately following the third round, complete cardio-burst options for 90 seconds: running or jogging or marching in place; side shuffles; jumping jacks; or jump rope.

JEN JUJU: Are You Taking On Too Much Too Quickly?

One of the biggest mistakes we make in our workouts is trying to do too much, too soon—which is why I designed the routines here to be only 16 minutes long. Let's say you tell yourself, "For the month of January, I'm going to the gym five times a week." Well, what happens when you miss your third day because your child is sick? And the next day, something else happens? By then, you're telling yourself, "Ugh. Forget it. I'm failing."

Or let's suppose you actually accomplish your commitment to exercise five times a week, but you can't keep it up. Now you either think you're lazy or you begin to believe you don't have what it takes to keep it up.

None of this is true! Take your workouts and the expectation of your performance within them a day at a time, and I guarantee you'll rise to the occasion. Remember, days grow into weeks, weeks into months, and before you know it you will have set that guilt down and begun to honor your own rhythm.

DUMBBELL EXERCISES

A-1: Overhead Triceps Press

Stand tall with your feet shoulder width apart and hold one light dumbbell in each hand, or one heavier dumbbell with both hands. Lift the weights over your head until both arms are fully extended. The palms of your hands should be facing up toward the ceiling.

Keeping your arms close to your head, lower the weights slowly behind your head, with your elbows in and perpendicular to the floor, until your forearms touch your biceps. Then slowly lift the weights back up to the ceiling. Lower to complete one rep.

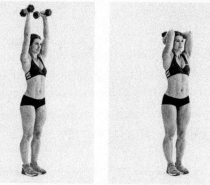

A-2: Overhead Triceps Squeeze

Stand tall with your feet together. With one light dumbbell in each hand, hold a 90-degree elbow position behind your head. With your chin up and shoulders back, push your hands into the weights and squeeze your elbows toward the center without allowing your arms to mobilize or straighten. Each squeeze is literally a pulse—less than 1 second long for one rep.

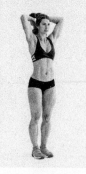

B-1: Side Laterals

Stand tall with your feet side by side and grasp a light to moderate dumbbell in each hand. Hold the dumbbells at your sides, with your palms facing inward. Slowly lift the dumbbells up, arms straight, to shoulder level in a T position. Slowly lower the weights to the starting position to complete one rep.

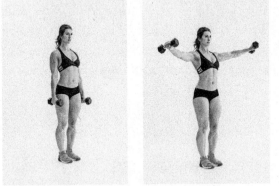

B-2: Arnold Presses

Stand tall with your feet side by side. Grasp a light to moderate dumbbell in each hand. Hold the two dumbbells in front of you at about upper chest level with your palms facing your body and your elbows bent. Now, raise the dumbbells as you rotate the palms of your hands until they are facing forward. Continue lifting the dumbbells until your arms are extended above your head in a straight-arm position. After a 1-second pause at the top, begin to lower the dumbbells to the original position by rotating the palms of your hands back toward you to complete one rep.

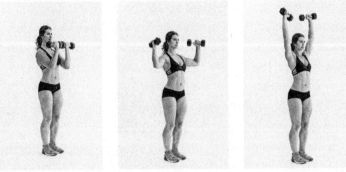

C-1: Reaching Forward Lunge

Stand tall and grasp light to moderate dumbbells in both hands, holding them at your sides, with your palms facing inward. Place your feet in a staggered position, with your left foot forward.

Bend your left leg deeply, lean in with your back straight, and extend the dumbbells all the way past your knees to the point of tapping the ground on either side of your left leg (if you can).

Then press back to the starting position using your core. Your back leg will bend very little; this exercise is all about the front leg working. Do 15 seconds with the left leg forward, then turn 180 degrees and do the remaining 15 seconds with the right leg forward to complete one rep.

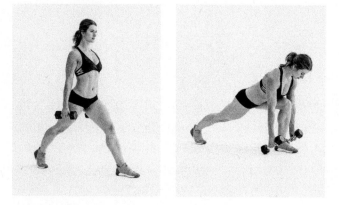

C-2: Alternating Snatch

Begin with your feet slightly wider than shoulder width apart. Place a light to moderate dumbbell between your feet. Looking out 4 feet in front of you, squat down only as far as it takes to grab the handle of the dumbbell with your left hand and forcefully push upward out of this position, generating as much power as you can in your lower back to heave the weight vertically up and above your head, palms facing forward. Keep the weight as close to your body as you can and do not swing the weight.

Return the dumbbell down the same path on which you brought it up, then lower your hips until the dumbbell once again makes contact with the floor. Repeat using your right hand to complete one rep.

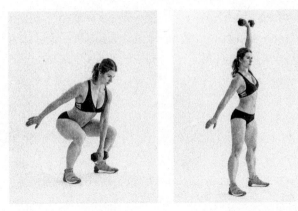

THE 16-MINUTE DUMBBELL ROUTINE

To complete the routine, perform Sequences A, B, and C consecutively.

SEQUENCE A

Complete three rounds of the following; try to increase the number of reps each cycle:

A-1: Overhead Triceps Press: Do as many reps as you can in 30 seconds.

A-2: Overhead Triceps Squeeze: Do as many reps as you can in 30 seconds.
Rest for 30 seconds.

Immediately following the third round, complete cardio-burst options for 90 seconds: running or jogging or marching in place; side shuffles; jumping jacks; or jump rope.

SEQUENCE B

Complete three rounds of the following; try to increase the number of reps each cycle:

B-1: Side Laterals: Do as many reps as you can in 30 seconds.

B-2: Arnold Presses: Do as many reps as you can in 30 seconds.
Rest for 30 seconds.

Immediately following the third round, complete cardio-burst options for 90 seconds: running or jogging or marching in place; side shuffles; jumping jacks; or jump rope.

SEQUENCE C

Complete three rounds of the following; try to increase the number of reps each cycle:

> **C-1: Reaching Forward Lunge:** Do as many reps as you can in 30 seconds.

> **C-2: Alternating Snatch:** Do as many reps as you can in 30 seconds.
> *Rest for 30 seconds.*

Immediately following the third round, complete cardio-burst options for 90 seconds: running or jogging or marching in place; side shuffles; jumping jacks; or jump rope.

BARBELL EXERCISES

A-1: Reverse Curls

Stand tall with your feet shoulder width apart. Take an overhand grip on a barbell, holding it with your arms down by your sides. Flex your elbows and slowly curl the bar up toward your chest and shoulders. Slowly lower the bar to the starting poistion at the top of your thighs to complete one rep.

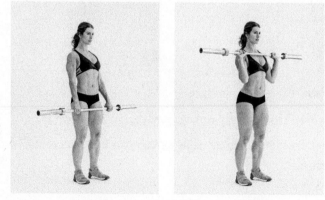

A-2: Back Squats

Stand tall with your feet slightly wider than shoulder width. Place the bar on your upper back with your hands just outside your shoulders.

Keep your head up at all times and maintain a fairly straight back as you bend your knees and sit back with your hips. Continue moving down until your hamstrings touch your calves. Slowly return to the starting position to complete one rep.

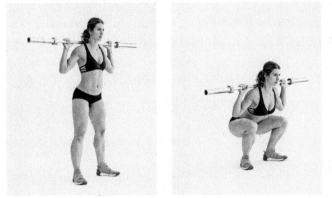

B-1: Stiff-Legged Deadlift

Stand tall with your feet slightly inside your shoulders with the barbell in your hands resting at your front thighs. With a slight bend in your knees, reach your hips back so that you're bending forward, and slightly lower the barbell along the top of your thighs and down 3 to 5 inches past your knees. Keep your chin tucked. Squeeze your booty and slowly return to the starting position, once again tracing the bar along your body without rounding your back to complete one rep.

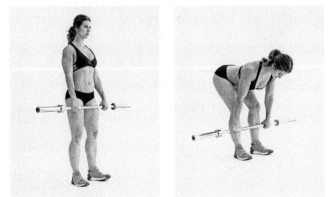

B-2: Sumo Deadlift High Pulls

Stand tall with your feet wider than shoulder width (sumo style), with your toes pointed outward.

Hold the barbell in front of you, with a slightly narrowed overhand grip on the bar. Lower your body slowly to the ground by bending your knees, allowing their trajectory to reach over toward your toes. Open up your chest and press your weight into your heels and the sides of your feet.

Stand back up, with the bar creating ground force, and accelerate the barbell into a high pull position, reaching your elbows above your collarbones and keeping your hands midchest. Return the bar to the starting position to complete one rep. *Note:* When using just the barbell (without weights), start with it just below your knees.

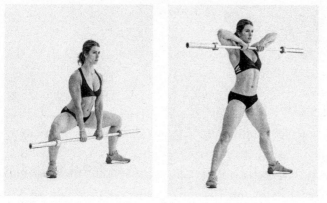

C-1: 90-Degree Focus Row/"No Swing Row"

Stand tall with your feet hip width apart and take an overhand grip on the barbell.

Bend over into a 90-degree position (or as close to that as you can get) with your arms extended. While keeping a straight back and connected core, slowly and consistently pull the bar all the way up until it touches just below your chest but above your belly button. Do not swing the barbell. Return to the starting position to complete one rep.

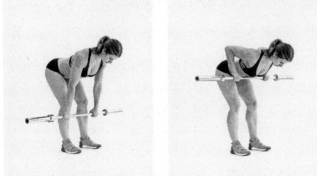

C-2: Front Squat to Press

Stand tall with your feet just outside shoulder width apart. Place the barbell in your front rack position, with the barbell across your collarbones and shoulders and your palms facing upward.

Keep your elbows forward, chest up, and back straight as you drop your hips down and back. Create the sensation of dragging your heels together as you stand up with the bar.

Do not drop your elbows and do not round your back as you do this. Once your legs are fully extended, allow momentum to build from the lower half of your body into your arms as you press the barbell above your head. Return to the starting position to complete one rep.

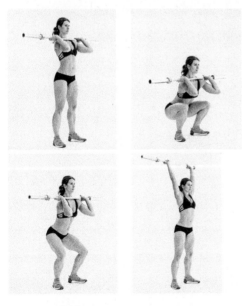

THE 16-MINUTE BARBELL ROUTINE

To complete the routine, perform Sequences A, B, and C consecutively.

SEQUENCE A

Complete three rounds of the following; try to increase the number of reps each cycle:

A-1: Reverse Curls: Do as many reps as you can in 30 seconds.

A-2: Back Squats: Do as many reps as you can in 30 seconds.
Rest for 30 seconds.

Immediately following the third round, complete cardio-burst options for 90 seconds: running or jogging or marching in place; side shuffles; jumping jacks; or jump rope.

SEQUENCE B

Complete three rounds of the following; try to increase the number of reps each cycle:

B-1: Stiff-Legged Deadlift: Do as many reps as you can in 30 seconds.

B-2: Sumo Deadlift High Pulls: Do as many reps as you can in 30 seconds.
Rest for 30 seconds.

Immediately following the third round, complete cardio-burst options for 90 seconds: running or jogging or marching in place; side shuffles; jumping jacks; or jump rope.

SEQUENCE C

Complete three rounds of the following; try to increase the number of reps each cycle:

C-1: 90-Degree Focus Row/"No Swing Row": Do as many reps as you can in 30 seconds.

C-2: Front Squat to Press: Do as many reps as you can in 30 seconds.
Rest for 30 seconds.

Immediately following the third round, complete cardio-burst options for 90 seconds: running or jogging or marching in place; side shuffles; jumping jacks; or jump rope.

MEDICINE BALL EXERCISES

(Use a 14-inch padded ball, 6 to 10 pounds.)

A-1: Chest Pass (to a Wall or a Partner)

Stand tall with the ball touching your chest, your elbows wide, with palm and finger pad pressure on the ball.

Extend your arms all the way out in front of you and release the ball. After it is returned to you, bring it all the way back to your chest again to complete one rep. These reps should cycle rather quickly.

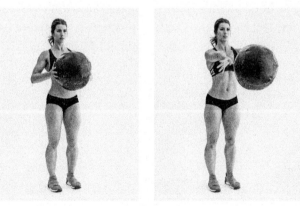

A-2: Overhead Pass (to a Wall or a Partner)

Stand tall with the ball in your hands and behind your head, with your elbows bent in a 90-degree starting position. Extend your arms forward and let the ball leave your hands in a relatively straight line. (I'm not looking for height on this but a directed pass.)

With your hands waiting over your head to receive the ball, catch it alone on your triceps and core to decelerate the ball's movement, returning to the start position to complete one rep.

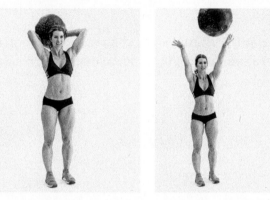

B-1: Right Kneeling Rotational (to a Wall or a Partner)

Start with your knees side by side (about 8 inches between them), with your heels together behind you. Swing the ball back to your left hip, keeping your eyes and shoulders aligned with the ball.

Next, orbit the ball across your body, following through with velocity and speed, to release the ball all the way to the wall or to your partner to the right of you. Once the ball comes back to you, swing the ball back to your left hip in the starting position to complete one rep. Cycling these reps should go rather quickly.

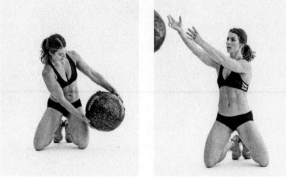

B-2: Left Kneeling Rotational (to a Wall or a Partner)

This exercise is identical to the previous one; however, the ball goes back to your right hip and you release it on the left side to complete one rep.

C-1: Weighted Knee Strikes

Lie on the ground with your legs straight and the ball between your hands above your head on the ground. Keeping your elbows open and finger pad pressure on the ball, bring the ball forward as you swiftly bring your left knee up to strike the ball. Return to the starting position before bringing up your right knee in the same action. Your head remains on the ground with your eyes on the ceiling *at all times*.

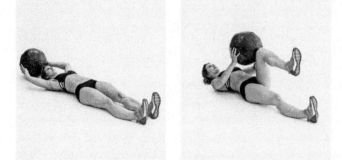

C-2: Squat to Vertical Toss

Stand tall with your feet just outside shoulder width apart and hold the medicine ball on your chest. Squat down, stand back up, and extend your arms, tossing the ball up vertically. Catch it to complete one rep.

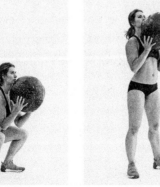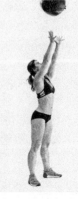

THE 16-MINUTE MEDICINE BALL ROUTINE

To complete the routine, perform Sequences A, B, and C consecutively.

SEQUENCE A

Complete three rounds of the following; try to increase the number of reps each cycle:

A-1: Chest Pass (to a Wall or a Partner): Do as many tosses as you can in 30 seconds.

A-2: Overhead Pass (to a Wall or a Partner): Do as many tosses as you can in 30 seconds.
Rest for 30 seconds.

Immediately following the third round, complete cardio-burst options for 90 seconds: running or jogging or marching in place; side shuffles; jumping jacks; or jump rope.

SEQUENCE B

Complete three rounds of the following; try to increase the number of reps each cycle:

B-1: Right Kneeling Rotational (to a Wall or a Partner): Do as many reps as you can in 30 seconds.

B-2: Left Kneeling Rotational (to a Wall or a Partner): Do as many reps as you can in 30 seconds.
Rest for 30 seconds.

Immediately following the third round, complete cardio-burst options for 90 seconds: running or jogging or marching in place; side shuffles; jumping jacks; or jump rope.

Complete three rounds of the following; try to increase the number of reps each cycle:

> **C-1: Weighted Knee Strikes:** Do as many reps as you can in 30 seconds.
>
> **C-2: Squat to Vertical Toss:** Do as many reps/tosses as you can in 30 seconds.
> *Rest for 30 seconds.*

Immediately following the third round, complete cardio-burst options for 90 seconds: running or jogging or marching in place; side shuffles; jumping jacks; or jump rope.

ISOMETRIC TO PLYOMETRIC EXERCISES

A-1: Wall Sit

Stand tall with your feet shoulder width apart. Press your shoulders and hips against a wall. Slide down until your knees are horizontal to the floor. Extend your arms straight out in front of you. Hold this position as long as you can.

A-2: Broad Jumps

With your feet together and some space in front of you, jump forward, landing softly and evenly on your feet. As you get more confident in this movement, you can extend the distance you jump.

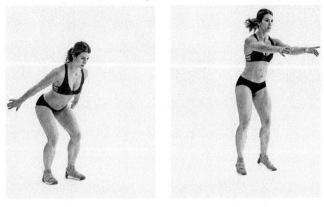

B-1: Midrange Push-up Hold

You can do this move on the ground, on an elevated bench, or leaning into a wall. With your hands 6 to 8 inches outside your shoulders, start in a solid plank position. Sink down into your push-up only 4 to 8 inches and hold for 30 seconds for one rep; if you fall out, shake your arms and go back to push-up position until the time is up.

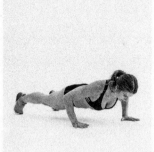

B-2: Springing Push-ups

You can do this move on the ground, on an elevated bench, or leaning into a wall. With your hands 6 to 8 inches outside your shoulders, start in a midrange push-up position. Press up and off the surface you're on, creating a moment of hang time in the air, and then return to the midrange push-up position to complete one rep.

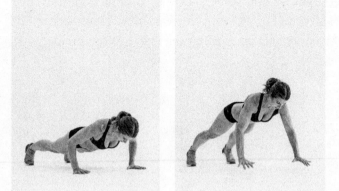

C-1: 3-Second Tempo Squats

Stand tall with your feet just outside shoulder width apart and your hands behind your head. Take 3 seconds to descend into your full squat position, pause for 1 second, and stand back up to complete one rep. Keep your eyes up and your torso vertical.

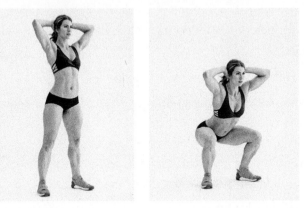

C-2: Squat Jumps/Box Jumps

Stand tall with your feet hip width apart and with your hands behind your head. Sink down into a squat position. As you come back up, ascend through the top of your squat into a jump, with your arms raised straight up above your head. As you grow more confident in this movement, transition from a hop, to a bigger jump, and then to your highest effort.

When you're ready, you can jump onto a box. Be sure to focus on clearing the height of the box, as well as landing softly, before you progress higher.

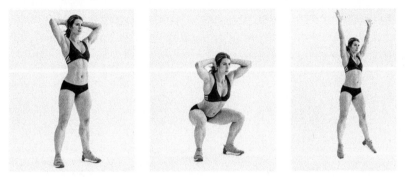

THE 16-MINUTE ISOMETRIC TO PLYOMETRIC ROUTINE

To complete the routine, perform Sequences A, B, and C consecutively.

SEQUENCE A

Complete three rounds of the following; try to increase the number of reps each cycle:

A-1: Wall Sit: Hold this position for 30 seconds.

A-2: Broad Jumps: Do as many jumps as you can in 30 seconds.
Rest for 30 seconds.

Immediately following the third round, complete cardio-burst options for 90 seconds: running or jogging or marching in place; side shuffles; jumping jacks; or jump rope.

SEQUENCE B

Complete three rounds of the following; try to increase the number of reps each cycle:

B-1: Midrange Push-up Hold: Execute this move and hold for 30 seconds.

B-2: Springing Push-ups: Do as many reps as you can in 30 seconds.
Rest for 30 seconds.

Immediately following the third round, complete cardio-burst options for 90 seconds: running or jogging or marching in place; side shuffles; jumping jacks; or jump rope.

SEQUENCE C

Complete three rounds of the following; try to increase the number of reps each cycle:

C-1: Second Tempo Squats: Do as many reps as you can in 30 seconds.

C-2: Squat Jumps/Box Jumps: Do as many jumps as you can in 30 seconds.
Rest for 30 seconds.

Immediately following the third round, complete cardio-burst options for 90 seconds: running or jogging or marching in place; side shuffles; jumping jacks; or jump rope.

COMBINATION #1 EXERCISES

These exercises use a variety of equipment.

A-1: L Shoulder Raise

Stand tall with your feet shoulder width apart, and grasp light to moderate dumbbells in your hands. Keep your core engaged and soften your knees. Raise one arm out to your side, while raising the other up to the front, creating an L with your arms.

The top of the movement is just above shoulder height. Return to the starting position and repeat on the other side to complete a rep.

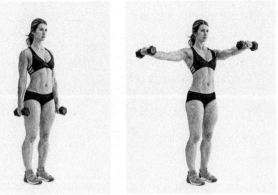

A-2: Rear Deltoid Press

Stand tall with your feet shoulder width apart, and grasp light to moderate dumbbells in your hands. Hinge forward from your waist at a 45-degree angle, with your arms extended and hanging just below your chest. Using the back of your shoulders and the small muscles between your shoulder blades (rhomboids), lift the dumbbells up and backward into a fly position. Return to the starting position to complete one rep.

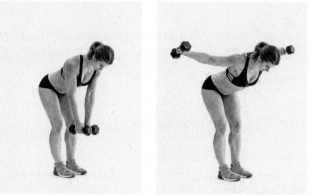

B-1: Walking Lunges

Stand tall and hold a barbell in front of you at the top of your chest, just under your neck. (You can also hold it on your back at the top of your shoulders.)

Step forward with the left leg and bend it into a lunge position. Bring the back leg forward and stand up. Lunge forward in the same manner with the right leg. Keep alternating legs and walking forward.

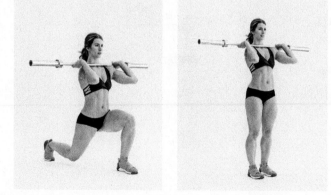

B-2: Lateral Hops/Jumps

Starting and landing on two feet, hop or jump over a line back and forth. As you get more confident, jump over a barbell, a bench, or even a box.

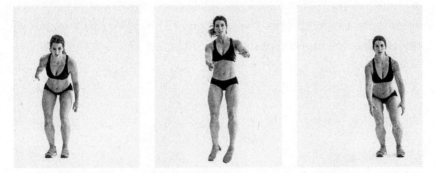

C-1: Banded Alternating Triceps T Press

Stand tall with your feet shoulder width apart and place your hands directly on the resistance band itself; do not hold the handles.

With moderate to light tension, extend both your arms out into a T position. With control, bend one elbow to a 90-degree angle, pausing for just a moment and then extending it back out to your T position. Repeat the same movement on the opposite side to complete a rep.

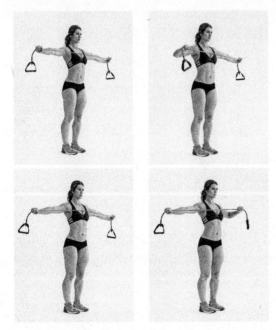

C-2: Banded Rhomboid Pulse

Stand tall with your feet shoulder width apart, holding the resistance band in the same T position as in the previous exercise, with arms extended and reaching sideways. Use the small muscles in the middle of your back and behind your shoulders to pull your arms backward, holding for 1 second. This 1-second pulse should be 1 to 2 inches of slow, connected movement for one rep.

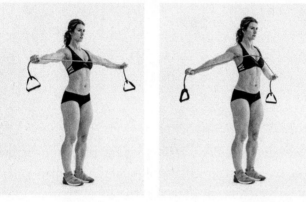

THE 16-MINUTE COMBINATION #1 ROUTINE

To complete this routine, perform Sequences A, B, and C consecutively.

SEQUENCE A

Complete three rounds of the following; try to increase the number of reps each cycle:

A-1: L Shoulder Raise: Do as many reps as you can in 30 seconds.

A-2: Rear Deltoid Press: Do as many reps as you can in 30 seconds.
Rest for 30 seconds.

Immediately following the third round, complete cardio-burst options for 90 seconds: running or jogging or marching in place; side shuffles; jumping jacks; or jump rope.

SEQUENCE B

Complete three rounds of the following; try to increase the number of reps each cycle:

B-1: Walking Lunges: Execute this walking action for 30 seconds.

B-2: Lateral Hops/Jumps: Do as many jumps as you can in 30 seconds.
Rest for 30 seconds.

Immediately following the third round, complete cardio-burst options for 90 seconds: running or jogging or marching in place; side shuffles; jumping jacks; or jump rope.

SEQUENCE C

Complete three rounds of the following; try to increase the number of reps each cycle:

C-1: Banded Alternating Triceps T Press: Do as many reps as you can in 30 seconds.

C-2: Banded Rhomboid Pulse: Do as many reps as you can in 30 seconds.
Rest for 30 seconds.

Immediately following the third round, complete cardio-burst options for 90 seconds: running or jogging or marching in place; side shuffles; jumping jacks; or jump rope.

COMBINATION #2 EXERCISES

These exercises use a variety of equipment.

A-1: Push-ups (Full Range)

Begin in the plank position and lower your body to the ground. Raise your body back up with your back straight, or raise your chest up first, then your hips, in order to return to the plank position to complete one rep. Just be sure to cycle through a full range of motion during this exercise.

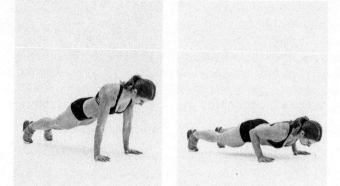

A-2: Single-Arm Dumbbell Deadlifts

Stand tall with your feet slightly wider than shoulder width. Hold a moderately heavy dumbbell in one hand.

Reach down and tap the ground with the dumbbell without rounding your back. As you start to stand up, explode up with force, allowing the dumbbell to transfer from one hand to the other. Repeat this sequence for one rep: tap the ground with the dumbbell, explode back up to the starting position, and transfer the dumbbell to the other hand. This is an exercise that takes coordination and requires constant movement.

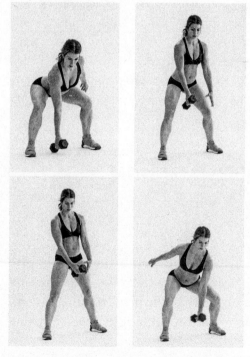

B-1: Weighted Push Press

Stand tall with your feet shoulder width apart, holding light to moderate dumbells at your collarbones, with your palms facing upward. (You can also use a barbell in a front rack position.)

Without dropping your elbows or rounding your back, dip your hips down, putting your weight on your butt and hamstrings. Pop your hips open and upward, allowing momentum to carry from the lower half your body into your arms, and press the weight straight over your head. Return to the starting position to complete one rep.

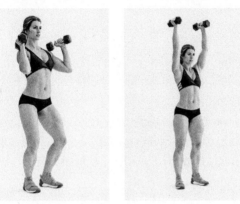

B-2: Pull-ups (Banded Simulation or Bar)

Loop a resistance band with handles over a rack that is taller than you in order to simulate a pull-up's range of motion.

Slightly pitch your hips back and extend your arms fully with your hands on the handles. Then with your neck and spine in alignment, use the muscles below your armpits (lats) and back to pull the handles all the way down to shoulder height. Release slowly back to the starting position to complete one rep.

If you're ready for a traditional pull-up, hang from a bar, using an overhand grip. Maintain a hollow body hold, with your lower back flat and abs drawn together as you pull your chin above the bar to complete one rep.

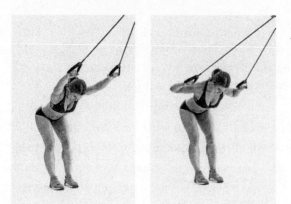

C-1: Weighted Front Squats

Stand tall with your feet just wider than shoulder width apart. Use light to moderate dumbbells (or a barbell) in your front rack position.

Keep your elbows forward and your rib cage vertical as you drop your hips down and back. Do not drop your elbows, and do not round your back. Create a sensation of dragging your heels together as you stand up to complete one rep

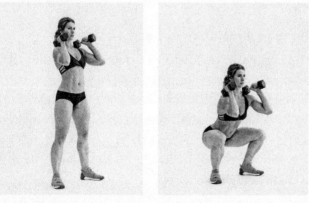

C-2: Squat Jumps/Box Jumps

Stand tall with your feet hip width apart and your hands behind your head. Sink down into a squat position. As you come back up, ascend through the top of your squat into a jump, with your arms raised straight up above your head. Return to the starting position to complete one rep. As you grow more confident in this movement, transition from a hop to a jump.

When you're ready, you can jump onto a box. Make sure you're starting and ending with your feet about 2 feet apart. Focus on clearing the height of the box, as well as landing softly, before you progress higher.

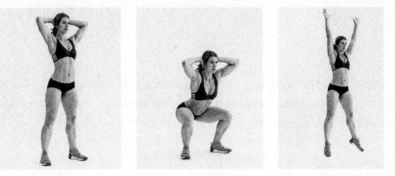

THE 16-MINUTE COMBINATION #2 ROUTINE

To complete the routine, perform Sequences A, B, and C consecutively.

SEQUENCE A

Complete three rounds of the following; try to increase the number of reps each cycle:

A-1: Push-ups (Full Range): Do as many reps as you can in 30 seconds.

A-2: Single-Arm Dumbbell Deadlifts: Do as many reps as you can in 30 seconds.
Rest for 30 seconds.

Immediately following the third round, complete cardio-burst options for 90 seconds: running or jogging or marching in place; side shuffles; jumping jacks; or jump rope.

SEQUENCE B

Complete three rounds of the following; try to increase the number of reps each cycle:

B-1: Weighted Push Press: Do as many reps as you can in 30 seconds.

B-2: Pull-ups (Banded Simulation or Bar): Do as many reps as you can in 30 seconds.
Rest for 30 seconds.

Immediately following the third round, complete cardio-burst options for 90 seconds: running or jogging or marching in place; side shuffles; jumping jacks; or jump rope.

SEQUENCE C

Complete three rounds of the following; try to increase the number of reps each cycle:

C-1: Weighted Front Squats: Do as many reps as you can in 30 seconds.

C-2: Squat Jumps/Box Jumps: Do as many jumps as you can in 30 seconds.
Rest for 30 seconds.

Immediately following the third round, complete cardio-burst options for 90 seconds: running or jogging or marching in place; side shuffles; jumping jacks; or jump rope.

How to Stay on Track

Getting yourself to cross the threshold of the gym's doors is often more challenging than the workout itself. I know we all have a million reasons as to why we "just can't make it to the gym today," but ironically all we need is one of those reasons to back out of it.

I realized the problem wasn't our lack of desire to be

there that kept us from getting to the gym but instead the self-imposed pressure of performance. We carry in our minds what our workouts need to look like or feel like to be effective or successful, so if we don't feel like we can attain that today, we talk ourselves out of going. But *why*?

Who cares if you ran last week but you need to walk today? Who cares if you choose a bike in the back row of your cycling studio because you don't have the energy to be on a bike in the front of the room like you usually do? Who cares if you usually train with heavier dumbbells but today you need lighter ones? Forget all that stuff and just do what you can do!

Why set these expectations and talk yourself out of going? Instead, let yourself off the hook and talk yourself *into* going. "I can walk as slow as I want in my warm-up mile." "I don't need to stay for the whole class, just hit the first forty-five minutes and bail." "I don't need to RX this workout or put my score up on the board." Simply get your body through the door.

But something cool almost always happens next. Once you begin to move, you start to open up to the workout and remember why you put exercise on your list in the first place. You start to feel good—great, even. Pretty soon, you're gaining momentum and your "just need to walk" self-talk for the workout graduates into jogging. You will naturally take on more and get a better session in than you'd even thought possible. And to think you were going to skip the gym—look what you would have missed!

If your body and mind happen to not make the turn that day, do not fret. Any movement is a victory on days like these, and don't think you have to exceed your prior performance and be a superstar every day in order to maintain your weight. Just be present and let yourself come to life through that workout. I'm telling you, get yourself through those gym doors and the rest will take care of itself.

PART 4

THE NEW, FIT YOU

CHAPTER 13

LESSONS FOR LIFELONG MAINTENANCE

A t a time when more than half of Americans regain the weight they lose, it is impossible to ignore the fallout of many diet plans. In all my years as a trainer, my job never ended in the gym. Staying connected to my clients through their (and my) personal highs and lows, kitchen catastrophes, and even bad dates held just as much weight for me as the few hours of gym time we had during the week.

Day after day, year after year, I saw every pattern, every default reaction, every missed opportunity, and began developing solutions for all of them. After ten years of collecting data and implementing solutions through trial and error, I have done the reps, and the years of success from my clients speak volumes about our findings.

My clients knew I was committed to their overall life success, and in our time together they learned how to commit to it, too. To feel seen and heard is critical to a person feeling relevant and worthy. I have poured my everything into this book because that is exactly the way I feel about you. You are so deserving of my support as well as a real solution. So in this chapter, I have decided to share with you the fruits of my labor, including all the maintenance protocols that will keep you tapped in to the success you've earned here. In addition, all of the recipes in this book can be used going forward, no matter what personality type you are. Follow these guidelines when it comes to your everyday meals, and continue to follow the eating schedule that works best for you.

Welcome to my inner circle.

LIFER TOOLS

Long-term maintainers have created patterns in their daily lives that support successful maintenance. Put another way, they've set their lives up for success. Here are some examples:

- They keep food logs or journals of what they eat so their food habits are real, written down in black and white. It's gratifying to look back on successful days, but there's also no hiding from bad ones. If my clients have a rough week, I encourage them to spend some time thinking through what went on around those meals, thinking back to why they overindulged so they can use it as a learning experience and exhibit control the next time that scenario arises.

- They set aside time over a weekend to prep for the week ahead. Personally, I always have fruit that is washed and cut. I roast a full tray of veggies for the week. I boil eggs for my snacks and make sure I have a lot of healthy grab-and-go snacks around. When you invest that small bit of time thinking about your food, your entire week becomes more executable. If you know there will be an executive meeting over lunch, for example, request a healthy salad. But if there's nothing acceptable, pack your own food. This isn't a big deal, so don't make it one! Also, don't allow yourself to go anywhere without your water bottle and a little Jen-approved nosh. Being prepared will keep you from falling into those poor-food-choice potholes, and instead will allow you to navigate around them because you've given yourself the upper hand.

- They have the tools to prep: steamer, slow cooker, nonstick cookware, blender or food processor—everything it takes to prepare easy, healthy meals. They also have plastic containers, plastic wrap, and microwavable containers for storing their food—even entire meals—so they can just pop them in the microwave for a fast dinner, as well as a personal lunch cooler they can take with them to store perishables and foods that need refrigeration on the days when there's no end in sight.

Bottom line, they've got their kitchen set up on autopilot to remove any variables that could potentially veer them off their healthy course.

- They develop little eating rules that keep them on track. Take my friend Beth, for example. On Friday nights, she orders her favorite pizza. No matter how hungry she is or how great the temptation, she never eats the whole pie. Just two to three pieces, and she throws in the towel. In a way, I think knowing she'll get to order pizza again the next week helps her stay so strong in her resolve, and there's a really cool element to that. Stop eating like you'll *never* get to have dessert again, or pizza, or soda. There will always be more opportunities to eat yummy foods again.

- They are good stress managers. No one gets a pass from tension at work, with family, or over finances. We all have stress in our lives. The key to managing it is how you respond to it. Identify your stress reliever in an activity or movement that is meditative for you. Too often I see folks eating as a response to stress, and it's no surprise because stress boosts your levels of the appetite-stimulating hormone cortisol, so you're already vulnerable. My most successful stress managers choose exercise; it dissipates cortisol, plus it has a mood-lifting effect on your entire body. So instead of reaching for the refrigerator door, reach for your tennis shoes and get movin'.

SLEEP AND SHRINK

Want to keep your weight off? . . . Then head to bed.

Like healthy food and good hydration, quality sleep is one of the three foundational pillars that optimize your body's ability to metabolize calories and fat—I'm talking six to eight hours of quality sleep a night. This is a nonnegotiable for me, and it shows up in my energy, yes, but my slim waistline, too. If you're sleep-deprived, you're more likely to put on pounds; it's really that cut-and-dry.

Every two years for sixteen years, the landmark Nurses Health Study looked at health data from more than 68,000 women ages forty to sixty-five, including information on their sleep habits and body weight. On average, nurses who slept five hours a night were 32 percent more likely to experience a weight gain of thirty-three pounds or greater, and 15 percent more likely to become obese, compared with those who slept seven hours a night.

Why is this? The amount and quality of sleep affects two hormones that regulate appetite and metabolism: leptin and ghrelin. Leptin is a hormone that suppresses appetite by making us feel full and satisfied after eating. Ghrelin is a hormone that stimulates appetite.

With sleep deprivation, levels of leptin dip, while ghrelin levels rise. With both hormones out of balance, there's an increase in appetite along with elevated cravings for sweets, salty foods, and starchy foods like bread and pasta. You'll be asking for nightly meals of buttered garlic bread with fettuccine Alfredo!

And, when people are tired from too little sleep, they don't feel like exercising, making those extra pounds even more accessible. Lack of sleep disrupts other hormones such as cortisol, insulin, and growth hormone, and this can trigger a desire for high-calorie foods.

We don't look at sleep as nourishment, but we should. It is the only time in which your body can work with the nutrients it receives during the day, in order to recover and repair overnight. So if you're not getting enough sleep or not getting quality sleep, your body's never able to truly heal itself and recharge. Your metabolism isn't optimal, your muscles aren't recovering, and you're not living and moving the way you should.

Let's get cozy: here are a few simple suggestions to help you get rested and stabilize your weight goal:

- Create an open environment in your bedroom—remove excess clutter and mess.
- Make sure your bedding is clean and comfortable.
- Use soothing scents, such as lavender oil on your pillows or scented candles.
- Sip a cup of calming tea before bedtime. Chamomile, lavender, valerian root, and passionflower teas work wonderfully.

- Do not use cell phones, TVs, and tablets for at least forty-five minutes before bedtime. These devices emit light of all colors, but the blue light in particular disrupts sleep. Blue light prevents the release of melatonin, a hormone associated with nighttime sleepiness.

HOLD THE LINE

We all have a baseline weight we'd like to maintain, but we all need to also set a nonnegotiable limit for ourselves—a weight that you absolutely will not exceed. This is an individual conversation to have with yourself that sets off your private alarm system when your weight drifts up out of your healthy range. Its purpose is to bring attention to the drifting and not allow eight pounds to turn into twenty, then thirty, and so on. The drift can be from the holidays or a vacation or even just a very busy couple of months.

Let me use myself as an example. My walk-around weight is 143 pounds, but my "line" is 150 pounds. If I hop on the scale and see it settling at 148 or above, I know that it's time to rein in the loose eating and get back in flow with my morning workouts. In your case, this is the signal to get straight back on your personalized meal plan. It's yours for life, after all, so lean in to it when you need my help to level you out.

I'd also like to add that monitoring your weight on the scale has been scientifically proven to keep you in range of your ideal weight. Numerous studies conducted by the prestigious National Weight Control Registry—a research study that gathers information from people who have successfully lost weight and kept it off—found that "weight maintainers" frequently weigh themselves to stay at their goal weights.

Scale-hopping doesn't have to become a professional sport; there is a clear relationship between frequent weighing and keeping weight off, so do it often to keep yourself in line.

EMBRACE YOUR SHAPE

I can't tell you how many times I've felt pressure from the "thin is in" trend and the criticism that I am too muscular and don't have a desirable appearance. For years, my desire to "fit in" far outweighed my desire to discover my own way of doing things in a healthy way . . . especially when it came to my body image. That is, until I learned to embrace my shape.

Some women are naturally built thinner, smaller. That is their genetic predisposition, and for them to be thin isn't unhealthy but their body's optimal state. The difference is when someone who is not of that predisposition compromises their health in order to achieve their "ideal body image." If you try to cram your square-peg, genetically given shape into a round hole, you're going to gradually erode your health and fitness. In my case, why would I want to give up my quality of life just to be less muscular?

As you identify your personality and finally find a program that "fits" you, it's important that you still remember to embrace your own body. Don't settle for someone else's construct of beauty. The only person who should set the expectation for what you want to look like is *you*. So as you quickly drop pounds and begin to feel reenergized, embrace the progress and don't compare yourself to some arbitrary "ideal" look.

YOUR DIET QUESTIONS, SIMPLIFIED

The biggest advantage of working with me? I know the problems you'll face before you even see them coming. That's the benefit of years of working with clients on a personalized level. While Chapter 3 was all about the basics, this section is designed to help you anticipate and troubleshoot different questions, problems, and concerns that could occur on the plan. Consider this just one more roadblock removed on your journey to the body you want and deserve.

#BODYTALK

We have already established how unique you are in psyche and behavior, but what about your body? Your body is talking to you all the time, and you probably don't even know it. Pain, discomfort, energy shifts—these are all ways that it tries to get information to you. So if you truly started to listen, what would it be telling you?

The conversations will differ, based on our heredity and individual sensitivities, but here's an example:

"Okay, Jen . . . you can ignore me all you want. But I'm going to make your eyes puffy, have you feeling sleepy all day, and throw in a headache on top of that . . . unless you give me more water today."

Here, my body is using physical signs and discomfort to communicate that I'm short on my fluids for the day. This is a pretty simple scenario, but it's remarkable when you think about how smart your body is. Not only does it never take a day off, but it knows us better than we know ourselves. It knows that water's job isn't just to quench your thirst but to hydrate your body, lubricate your organs, help firm your skin (including under your eyes), and maintain metabolism.

Another clear example of how our body talks to us relates to food. If you don't get enough, you may feel weak and shaky. If you overeat, you may also feel sick. It's the same with exercise. If you get the right amount, you feel energized, your mood is bright, and you're more alert.

It's also important to have a clear understanding of what kinds of foods your body digests well. For example, ask yourself these two questions after your meals:

1. Do you feel bloated and sleepy?
2. Do you lack appetite for three or more hours after a meal?

If you said yes, this signals to me that something in what you've eaten is not optimal in your system, so you're struggling to digest it and should consider other food options. On the other hand, if you feel energized, alert, and hungry within a couple hours after your meal, you're on track and you know to keep those foods in your nutrition scheme.

I stumbled into this whole way of thinking five years ago over a simple bowl of rice. I was on this wild rice medley kick because it was steamed fresh daily at this amazing little Japanese store by my home. It was delicious and a perfect healthy grab-and-go after working all day. I would usually have about a cup of the rice with some fish and a green veggie. A solid, healthy meal, if you ask me. But it seemed like I was always a bit distended after having rice, and the following morning I'd not wake up hungry like I normally do. Ultimately, I just chalked it up to my Chicago upbringing and eating too fast and too late.

But then one day, it happened. Forced to break my routine because I arrived at the store too late and was met with an empty rice steamer, I threw a sweet potato in my cart to go with my standard fish and a green veggie. Dinner came and went, and looking back I was too tired to notice much of anything. But when I woke up the next day, it was like gravity had left the room. I woke up ravenous. I literally had more ab definition than I did the day before (goodbye, bloated belly!). I'd also never realized how groggy I'd been in the mornings—because of how clear-headed I now felt that morning.

It finally hit me. My body does better with the sweet potatoes than it does with rice, even though both are healthy, nutritious foods. One just digests better in my system than the other. So do I not eat rice now? Almost never. From time to time, I'll sneak in a little with my sushi, but now that I know how good I can feel, I opt to keep it out of my diet.

Your elevated awareness of your body is what I'm asking for. Pay attention to what I've already listed, but also watch for changes in your skin, sleep quality, and, on an awkward note, even feedback from below the belt. Are you consistently gassy or experiencing sporadic bowel movements? Whether you answer yes or no, this is major feedback for you!

When you consume food your body can't tolerate, like dairy products if you are lactose intolerant, wheat products if you are gluten sensitive, or other foods to which you might be allergic, it's going to show up. Or this could even just be food your body has difficulty breaking down, like rice for me.

Pay attention to your food and how it makes you feel. If something doesn't agree with you, play around with removing it and be open to discovering substitutes that improve your system, not bog it down.

The big takeaway is that when you make it easier for your body to do its job, you're able to metabolize and drop pounds more effectively, so let's do your body a favor and become a better listener.

HOW SHOULD I HANDLE RESTAURANTS OR TAKEOUT?

As part of your plan, you may eat out one night *each* week, as long as you do so under the following parameters:

- Don't go to dinner starving. Have a healthy mini snack right before you go.
- Choose a healthy protein, such as whitefish, salmon, steak filet, white meat chicken (no skin), shrimp, or scallops.
- If you choose to have an alcoholic beverage, consider it your starch intake for the meal. Don't double-portion yourself on carbs. In other words, when booze is your carb for the night—no bread basket, potato, sweet potato, rice, or quinoa.
- Eat nothing fried.
- Have the salad dressing and sauces served on the side. (Dip your fork in the dressing or sauce, then spear your food. Do this for each bite.)
- Be accountable for your portions. Identify your correct portions using my plate example (see page 46) and leave behind whatever is beyond that.

WHAT'S A FOOD YOU LOVE THAT MOST PEOPLE DON'T DISCUSS?

I'm a super fan of the superfoods spirulina and chlorella—two forms of green algae that are superior plant-based proteins and have far-reaching health benefits. In fact, the first thing I do in the morning is drink a tall glass of water with algae tablets, as a part of my breakfast. I've found that these supplements give me more energy, cleanse the body, and tame cravings. I haven't missed a day of taking them in the last six years because I literally feel that good on them.

Spirulina is packed with vitamins such as B1 (thiamine), B2 (riboflavin), B3 (nicotinamide), B6 (pyridoxine), B9 (folic acid), C, A, and E, and it contains the highest concentration of plant protein in the world. It is so nutritious that NASA astronauts and Olympic athletes have used it for decades.

In treadmill tests, people who consumed spirulina before their workout improved their performance and endurance compared with those taking a placebo. Other research found that spirulina helps eliminate metals and other toxins from the body.

My other algae friend, chlorella, has something spirulina doesn't: a substance called chlorella growth factor (CGF). Extracted from the nucleus of the chlorella cell, CGF is a complex of nutritive compounds that have medicinal properties. Both chlorella and CGF are believed to protect against cancer, heart disease, and immune disorders. There are also theories that chlorella and CGF could help people lose weight, though the jury is still out on this one. Like spirulina, chlorella is also known to be a mild detoxifying agent that can help rid the body of heavy metals and toxins.

I KNOW THEY'RE IMPORTANT, BUT I DON'T LIKE VEGETABLES. ANY ALTERNATIVES?

Are veggies a big ick factor for you? We need to talk about this hate-vegetables thing. With veggies, you need to answer a simple question: Is it the taste or the texture that turns you off?

I used to hate asparagus, for example, because it would turn too mushy when cooked. I'd take a bite but could never quite get through it all the way, then couldn't chew it because it was so fibrous. Strips of the asparagus would stick in my teeth, or hang out of my mouth. Let's just say I knew what to avoid on date night.

Asparagus and I were done, but as a last-ditch effort, I tried a different way of cooking it—blanching—which means cooking in boiling water or in steam for a very short time, so that it is still raw and crispy. Blanching changed asparagus for me. I love it now! You can blanch with other veggies, too, such as broccoli, cauliflower, and Brussels sprouts. Broiling is another great option I stumbled upon for cooking veggies while still keeping them crisp.

If it's a taste thing, that's a little more serious. I have a client who hated broccoli and a lot of other veggies and just refused to eat them. So we had to get creative.

This client *loved* Buffalo wings (after all, who doesn't?), so I bought his favorite wing sauce, which was low in carbs and calories, and stir-fried vegetables with just a little water and a few tablespoons of the sauce. He's been eating his veggies like that and dropping weight ever since.

One additional tip is to chop up your vegetables into smaller pieces and lightly coat them with your favorite salad dressing. That's what I did with kale (yes, I used to hate it, too), and now kale is my friend.

One more piece of advice: go nuts with your veggies, especially greens, and eat them in unlimited portions. Green veggies contain lots of trace nutrients that get right into your blood, right into your physical body, right into your skin, and right into your muscle.

WHAT'S THE WORD ON LATE-NIGHT SNACKS?

Sorry, friends, no late-night snacks. A study published in the *American Journal of Physiology* in 2013 found that nighttime snacking increased total and LDL cholesterol (the artery-clogging type) and interfered with fat-burning, suggesting that eating at night changes fat metabolism and increases the risk of obesity. (Caveat: Anyone who has type 1 diabetes should indeed eat before bedtime, because it is important for blood sugar control overnight and even survival.)

For most people, nighttime eating—especially after eight p.m.—isn't a great idea. You're loading your stomach with calories at a time when your body is slowing down, and those calories won't get adequately burned off. If you absolutely must eat something later at night, choose pure protein. Eating a little protein before bedtime not only boosts your metabolism while you sleep, but it may also increase your metabolism into the next day. For a good late-night snack, make yourself a small omelet with some veggies and a little cheese—or have some nuts, avocado, flaxseed, chicken, or fish.

I HAVE A SWEET TOOTH. DO YOU BELIEVE IN CHEAT DAYS?

In my mind, cheat days don't exist because I don't believe that you're cheating on anything! You are supposed to live fully and enjoy life, and I don't believe that eating perfectly brings that out in any of us. It's also difficult to have a system where you eat perfectly, then have one whole day where you cut loose, because unless you have extreme discipline like The Rock, it's just too hard to reset your body. By the time your system has recovered, that one day has turned into three entire days where your body could have been losing weight versus rebounding. In my experience, one healthy day of eating is the equivalent of three days going to the gym—so be careful not to trade three workouts for a lazy junk meal if it's not important to you.

I will say, though, every once in a while I'll go to Hooters or Portillo's when I travel through Chicago. Or I'll have a doughnut— preferably a chocolate long john. I don't assign them as cheats but rather as chosen indulgent moments, and you should have them, too! But choosing to eat well end-to-end, one day into the next, becomes a powerful asset; don't let too many indulgent moments take that power away from you.

WHAT SHOULD I DO WHEN WEIGHT LOSS STALLS?

DON'T OVERTHINK IT. First of all, your body really does want to be thin. It doesn't want to be fat and unhealthy. You must be patient with it as it drops pounds because you're finally giving it good food and regular exercise.

What may feel like a plateau is just your body losing at its own pace—maybe three pounds one week and one pound another week. Be patient with your body. Don't stress over not losing pounds. That stress will further slow down your weight loss, because stress causes your body to churn out fat-building cortisol. Relax. Be consistent with nourishment, hydration, and exercise, and your body will do its thing.

AFTERWORD: BEFORE YOU GO . . .

You. Are. Ready.

It is time to take ownership of your newfound knowledge, get into the driver's seat, and apply it to the rest of your life! You are armed with the information, momentum, and—just as important—the confidence to make decisions that will shape the way you fuel your body and your future.

At first, you will do this consciously, but later it will be effortless and enjoyable. (I promise!) You'll start functioning with more ease, and you'll surprise yourself with how much more you can take on. You have given yourself a fighting chance to build and create a sense of self and purpose. Most important, you'll realize you had what it took all along to live a healthy life.

It has taken courage to admit that you need to do something about your weight. To walk into a gym or a cardio class . . . peek at the scale . . . admit you're scared that you might fail—again—and look deeply into your own personality and make a change. Most consider this process a sign of weakness, when in reality it shows tremendous strength. I cannot express enough how proud I am of you for this.

Going forward, believe in yourself and in your purpose. Realize that you—and you alone—determine your relevance and have the power to create change. Embrace the choices you make, recognize their value, and no matter what your journey looks like, never underestimate your self-worth.

I know fear can distort reality and cloud your ability to move forward into the unknown. So if hard times return, come back to this book and recenter your mind-set, approach, and self-belief. Retake the assessment and see how you've shifted and grown. Take the time to recognize where you've become stronger and where you still need to improve. I wrote this book so that I can always be there for you to help you through the process, but you need to make sure that you are there for yourself, too.

In my last little hug to you, I want you to close this book knowing it's okay to bet on yourself and believe in your purpose. Own the realization that your joy, worth, and strength come from within. Remember, you determine if you're an afterthought, and you can also determine if you're a priority.

This is your life. It's time to make it yours and enjoy every second as if it's the only option.

Be the lion,

xx
You

ACKNOWLEDGMENTS

was a kid who didn't grow up with very much confidence, but whenever someone believed in me, they changed the course of my life. These impactful relationships didn't stop in my childhood. Through college, then later transitioning into life in Los Angeles and now in my career in television, I have held a sense of courage and passion that I could finally believe in because all of these people believed in me first. There are few greater feelings than being truly seen and heard and *accepted* for it. To be able to live and love and learn without judgment has been my privilege because the following people chose to use their lives investing in mine.

THANK YOU . . .

To my family, from generations before me and now after, for a foundation I will carry with me the rest of my life. Resilience, integrity, and heart are the pillars of who I am because of you. A special thanks to my siblings, Kristin and Erik, for nurturing the weird and wacky in me and making the garden plot fun because I was sharing the work with my two best friends. To my pops, for putting dumbbells in my hands, always letting me sing in car rides home (regardless of pitch), and nourishing seeds of courage within me. And to my mother, for teaching me what it was to truly be a strong woman, and how to live it.

To my dearest friends and mentors who sit in "my front row," from Chicago to KU to Los Angeles and now Boston. You are an extension of my family that lives no farther from my heart than they do.

I would not be able to thrive without your support; know that you are and will always be my brothers and sisters.

To my irreplaceable team at PMK, Nicole Perez and Alex Price; my agent and true renaissance woman, Andrea Barzvi, at Empire Literary; my remarkable Harmony team led by Diana Baroni, Michele Eniclerico, Julie Cepler, Stephanie Davis, Jules Horbachevsky, and Tammy Blake; Dr. Belisa Vranich for being my brainstorm buddy; Endemol Shine, NBC, and my *Biggest Loser* family, from our courageous contestants to producers to camera teams to audio to glam to our grips and beyond: You all may never quite understand how far your love and trust have taken me. Through the hardest times of this journey, it was your strength and friendship that fueled me, allowing me to become a better human being.

Finally, Adam Bornstein, words limit my ability to fully express my gratitude for you. Without you this book neither would have been started, nor would it have been finished. You challenged me to write out my stories and took the fear out of the process. Thank you for being my Clark Kent and my Superman.

In closing, I want to give an important shout-out to all of you on Team Jen on social media and beyond—you touch my life and make me better every single day. Without you being you, I could never be me.

REFERENCES

Boschmann, M., et al. 2003. "Water-induced thermogenesis." *Journal of Clinical Endocrinology and Metabolism* 88: 6015–19.

Cass R., and Sunstein, J. D. 2015. "Nudging smokers." *New England Journal of Medicine* 372: 2150–51.

Catenacci, V. A. 2014. "Dietary habits and weight maintenance success in high versus low exercisers in the National Weight Control Registry." *Journal of Physical Activity & Health* 11(8): 1540–48.

Chen, L., et al. 2009. "Reduction in consumption of sugar-sweetened beverages is associated with weight loss: the PREMIER trial." *American Journal of Clinical Nutrition* 89: 1299–1306.

Eckel, R. H. 2006. "Preventive cardiology by lifestyle intervention: opportunity and/or challenge?" Presidential address at the 2005 American Heart Association Scientific Sessions. *Circulation* 113: 2657–61.

Hammock, D. A. 2004. "Lose weight—without going hungry: tired of diets that leave your tummy rumbling? We've got the secret to staying slim while feeling full." *Good Housekeeping.* http://www.goodhousekeeping.com/health/diet-nutrition/advice/a23960/diet-no-hunger-hammock-0804/.

Kalafati, M., et al. 2010. "Ergogenic and antioxidant effects of spirulina supplementation in humans." *Medicine and Science in Sports and Exercise* 42: 142–51.

Markland, D. 1999. "Self-determination moderates the effects of perceived competence of intrinsic motivation in an exercise setting." *Journal of Sport and Exercise Psychology* 21: 350–60.

Mõttus, R., et al. 2013. "The associations between personality, diet and body mass index in older people." *Health Psychology* 32: 353–60.

Patel, S. R., et al. 2006. "Association between reduced sleep and weight gain in women." *American Journal of Epidemiology* 164: 947–54.

Pesta, D. H., and Samual, V. T. 2014. "A high-protein diet for reducing body fat: mechanisms and possible caveats." *Nutrition and Metabolism* 11: 53.

Prochaska, J. O., and DiClemente, C. C. 1992. "Stages of change in the modification of problem behaviors." *Progress in Behavioral Modification* 28: 183–218.

Prochaska, J. O., et al. 1992. "Attendance and outcome in a work site weight control program: processes and stages of change as process and predictor variables." *Addictive Behavior* 17: 35–45.

Reimer, R. A., et al. 2013. "Changes in visceral adiposity and serum cholesterol with a novel viscous polysaccharide in Japanese adults with abdominal obesity." *Obesity* 21: E379–87.

Schusdziarra, V., et al. 2011. "Successful weight loss and maintenance in everyday clinical practice with an individually tailored change of eating habits on the basis of food energy density." *European Journal of Nutrition* 50: 351–61.

Suarez, E. C., et al. 1998. "Neuroendocrine, cardiovascular, and emotional responses of hostile men: the role of interpersonal challenge." *Psychosomatic Medicine* 60: 78–88.

Sullivan, S., et al. 2007. "Personality characteristics in obesity and relationship with successful weight loss." *International Journal of Obesity* 31: 669–74.

Sutin, A. R., and Terracciano, A. 2015. "Personality traits and body mass index: modifiers and mechanisms." *Psychology and Health* 31: 259–75.

Sutin, A. R., et al. 2011. "Personality and obesity across the adult life span." *Journal of Personality and Social Psychology* 101: 579–92.

INDEX